THE SPIRIT OF THE MATTER

MYSORE STYLE ASHTANGA YOGA AND THE METAPHYSICS OF YOGA TĀRĀVALĪ

JOSH PRYOR

Warmth to my teacher Dan for persisting with me and reading my needs so well over the years he taught in Newcastle, and for bestowing the enormous favour of mentorship in those formative years of my teaching career.

Deepest gratitude to Rebecca and Jacqui for invaluable assistance from the very beginning of these ideas. Thanks as well to Yolanda and Helen for crucial assistance in crafting this work. Thanks to the generous community of students and teachers of Newcastle for providing the energetic domain needed to develop this book.

Salutations to Luke for the infinitudes of friendship through all my excursions.

Patañjali artwork on front cover: Melanie Mitchell
Illustrations within: Mathew Pryor
Photographs within: Cat Mead, Kate Binnie, Ash Wheelhouse, Dean Abraham

Published by Gorakhnath Pty Ltd

Second edition: August 2021
www.joshpryor.com.au

ISBN (Print): 978-0-6451211-0-0
ISBN (Digital): 978-0-6451211-1-7

FOR JACQUELINE
WITH EYES OF
THE BLACK STAG

TABLE OF CONTENTS

Note on Sanskrit terms and translations

Throughout this book you will find terms in the Sanskrit language. Sanskrit features pronunciation and grammar rules that are interesting to learn, but it takes time.

When a word is in italics, it means I have added all necessary diacritic marks (the lines and dots) so that the reader can begin building familiarity with these conventions.

Where a word is a proper noun or has been heavily Westernised, I have chosen to print it as normal English text with minimal diacritic markings. For example, the word *saṃskṛta* has been printed simply as "Sanskrit" throughout the text.

In other cases, I have chosen to keep words like *"anāhata"* in italics with full diacritics, in this case the bar over the second "a", indicating it is to be pronounced as a long vowel.

Furthermore, when the text Yoga Tārāvalī is being presented in chapter six, additional information is provided in [brackets] to help readers contextualise the phrases. In translating this text, I have used words that are faithful to the original while alive to the needs of students currently practicing.

PREFACE

Yoga is recognition of the higher Self

The practice of *yoga* in a way that considers a range of techniques, as is the case in Mysore style class settings, is the most effective tool for living a productive and grounded life while travelling along a clear path to the ultimate goal. That is, recognition of the higher Self.

The metaphysical reality espoused and realised by the great *yogin*-s is more than a romantic idea, more than an academic or philosophical pursuit, and much more than a historical ritual. It is a system of knowledge that empowers the individual to understand their place as the ultimate controller of their universe. It is a series of techniques which people can test for themselves and thereby know the truth.

While *yoga* as a general idea is widespread and popular, a rather substantial gulf remains between physical practices and the rest of the system of metaphysical enquiry, contemplation and concentration. People tend to do one or the other and thus achieve only a partial result. It is important to know that the two can be completely blended. A physical practice can be imbued with the highest form of spiritual knowledge, and the Mysore style environment facilitates this blending in a way unapproachable by more commercialised class formats.

The popular Ashtanga Vinyasa method of physical practice is intended to be combined with more esoteric components of *yoga*. This book will highlight the ancient Sanskrit text called Yoga Taravali, written by

Adi Shankara[1] — one of the greatest revolutionaries, writers, and *yogin*-s in the history of India. The creators of the Ashtanga Vinyasa Yoga system chose to wed it to this beautiful and concise *haṭha yoga* text.

While we have access to such Sanskrit texts and modern commentaries on them, the limitations of language result in only a partial revelation. Much study of Sanskrit is required to even begin to reveal the subtleties. In this book we will see how the complete blending of the physical and spiritual worlds are examined in the Mysore style setting.

We have a very clear opportunity and mandate to recognize the nature of reality and to play in the world in a way that awakens the intuitive and psychic faculties. It is a play that results in harmony, ecstatic experience, understanding of others, and control of one's own fate.

As a culture, we have imposed on ourselves for a long time a sense of limitation, an ingrained amnesia of the higher realities. Sometimes a fleeting glimpse is noticed. It usually occurs while sleeping, or out of the corner of the eye, and then half-remembered or forgotten altogether.

This process sometimes requires an eerie kind of courage. It can be terribly exciting, like standing at the edge of the water and aching to jump in, but feeling unprepared.

Great fun can be had in these threshold experiences. I remember camping with my old friends, all of us standing near a rope swing with a big drop down towards the river below. None of us were going to jump, but all of us really did want to have a go. No one was willing to walk away. It was an awkward stalemate.

---

[1] Written as Yoga Tārāvalī and Śaṅkarācārya using proper diacritic marks.

I was standing nearest the rope, and suddenly one of my friends gave me a big shove towards the water! My only choices in that moment were to either tumble down the embankment or jump and grab onto the rope and enjoy a big swing over the river.

I'm grateful he did that for me, gave me a push so that I had to do what I really wanted to do, even though it was scary.

It's this feeling of an exciting threshold that we need to watch for in order to grow in a naturally joyful manner. It is the sign that we are standing near the edge of our abilities, peeking out into a greater understanding, a bigger future, ready to learn something new.

This is a call to action. In this particular life, in this particular age of humankind, we can experience and live the realities that have been heretofore hidden from view.

We have everything we need. Let's go.

Introduction

Spring comes to the mountain top

The term "Mysore style" is used to denote a class format where several students can be in one room, each practicing at their own pace. They practice the poses and techniques that have been prescribed to them individually by their teacher. Mysore style classes are the most effective method of teaching large groups of students in a way that accommodates a wide range of ages and abilities, thus encouraging a lifelong practice.

This class format has been under-represented in the West since the explosion of a new form of commercial *yoga* class that spread in the 1980s, a "led" style of class that mimics group fitness classes that are found in gyms. In these classes all participants do the same thing at the same time as cued by an instructor.

The name Mysore style comes from the city of Mysuru in South India. So much of modern *yoga* came from this area. One type that developed in this region was Ashtanga Vinyasa Yoga, a series of postures and a practice method promulgated in the 20th century by several prominent teachers. The Mysore style teaching format is central to this flavour of *yoga*, which has come to be known simply as Ashtanga Yoga.

In a Mysore style class, everyone is taught one-on-one while sharing a group space. Students learn postures gradually according to their own needs and preferences, in concert with the assessment of their teacher. Every human body is unique and it is desirable to learn poses in a way that is tailored to suit the individual skeleton, physical fitness, and emotional temperament.

In Mysore style classes, difficult poses are given to a student only when they are ready to take on the new challenge. This style of teaching allows the sequence of moves to be so closely tailored to the individual that they can be balanced upon the leading edge of their ability at all times. Continuous flow is the aim, students take progressive steps into the unknown so that their capacity is gradually and joyfully increased.

In the historical context, Mysore style is actually not special — it is just the way *yoga* has always been taught. It is only in the last couple of decades, with the influx of *yoga* into the West, that there is a preponderance of the led class format. In this book, I will show that Mysore style classes are the most rational next step beyond led classes to allow the flourishing of each individual within a time-tested and safe framework.

For *yoga* teachers, Mysore style teaching environments offer a fantastic opportunity to facilitate joyful expansion and growth for their students. These classes offer something gripping and utterly educational for years to come.

The widespread use of the led class model in the West has resulted in a substantial uptake of *yoga* by the population, albeit with a relatively generalised method of teaching. This popularity is a wonderful thing for exposing the ideas of *yoga* to Western culture and preparing the ground for a more complete format.

It is easy to see why led classes are a commercially sensible way to run through *yoga* poses with large groups of people. The idea is to show people a sequence of postures covering a variety of movements without requiring much preparation. It is a formulaic and scalable way of giving people a taste of *yoga* and its benefits. In a led class, the instructor calls out poses to the group, gives general advice and motivational content.

When I teach led classes myself, I summarise the practice of *yoga* into a light-hearted and fun activity, where the objective is to do standard poses, bolstered by correct breathing. It is quite enjoyable for me, instructing groups in this fashion. It is nice to be helpful and uplifting in front of a group of eager people, to be a jovial instructor of a quasi-spiritual fitness class. It's very rewarding seeing people have a good time, and I have found it an opportunity to develop my own ability to encourage people to smile and laugh and relax in the moment.

When teaching Mysore style classes, the feeling is very different. Rather than being an extroverted figurehead of the group, the teacher is very much on the sidelines engaging the students one-on-one. Imagine a school classroom where all the students are at their desks working independently on their assignments and the teacher is walking around, tutoring, and checking their work.

When I first discovered Mysore style, as a student, I felt like I had hit the jackpot! Instead of being instructed as part of a group, I was now being coached and attended to one-on-one.

Instead of having to filter out the unneeded cues from the teacher and trying to glean the gems, I was able to enjoy peaceful movement at my own pace. I could ask for help when needed, and was being supervised by an expert whose sole focus was on helping to gradually improve my practice.

Among other things I was chuffed about the sheer sense of value for money. For the same class fee, I was now getting a personal lesson. What was I buying previously in all those led classes?

There is a point in a student's journey where it is necessary to step up into a more self-sufficient and self-motivated practice, under the tuition of an expert. Note that many people around the world start *yoga* in this traditional manner. This is the way *yoga* has been taught and practiced for a long, long time. This emphasis on self-authority is the reason for the truly transcendental experiences of the *yogin*-s of lore.

For those migrating from led classes, the motivation that was formerly projected from the instructor in an overt manner now comes from within you, and from the subtle influence of the other students in the room, who are also pursuing their own practice and having fascinating experiences.

Mysore style classes are a logical progression, the most obvious path to allow the complete flourishing of the individual within a dynamic and supportive framework. It is a practice unique in its scope, one that involves a blend of introversion and community, a sharing of quiet earnest aspiration and vulnerability. The creation of this environment has flow-on effects for the individual, the community, and the planet.

A Mysore style class can be daunting, even for confident people. I am quite sure that people can sense, in advance, the transformative effect that it will have on them. People hesitate to dive into Mysore style practice to a greater extent than led classes. They stand on the water's edge a little longer before jumping in.

In led classes you can be anonymous and blend into the crowd. You can allow your inner dialogue to be drowned out by the voice of the instructor. You know that no matter how difficult it gets you will soon be distracted by the next pose being delivered. Constant activity and variety characterise led classes and the required investment of conscious attention is relatively low.

A friend of mine is a successful real estate agency owner, very outgoing and confident. He recently revealed to me that he once attempted to come to a Mysore style class. He arrived at the studio, walked up the stairs, paused at the door… and walked back down to his car and drove off. This is remarkably common.

Nonetheless, Mysore style *yoga* offers things that are necessary for our species to flourish: new adventures, thrilling vulnerability, super-sensory awareness, stunning empathy, euphoric expansion, and breath-taking self-intimacy lie ahead.

1

AN ASHRAM FOR THE MODERN AGE

Closing the gap between the ideal and the ordinary

Once upon a time, humanity segregated spiritual seekers from regular people. Those people who wished, or were selected, to pursue spiritual callings were cloistered away in monasteries and ashrams while the rest of the population lived an ordinary life. Interactions between mystics and the populace occurred in varying degrees, but mostly, the search for the meaning of life was delegated to others. Perhaps we were busy, or afraid to tinker with underlying beliefs and assumptions. Not any longer.

The purpose of a classical ashram is to do spiritual practices while being supported by a teacher and a community of like-minded people. You do physical, meditative, mental, and emotional practices in a way that supports deep focus and concentration, attention across many domains, and persistent states of upliftment.

The same occurs in Mysore style classes; we perform postures, breathing, concentration, relaxation, and meditation in order to achieve joyous insight.

A Mysore style program offers an ashram experience for the modern age, a community space where empowered individuals gather to grow and share together. It is so bold as to increase our sense of both individuality and unity. It includes the paradoxical concept that we are at once unique and uniform. We are individualised entities that also exist as a single collective entity. Specialised fragments dancing as many different forms, and also as one whole form.

As the capacity for insight develops, more is seen and thus integrated. Blind spots are removed, empathy towards facets of one's self increases, and thus the subconscious becomes conscious.

So too does the world around us appear increasingly integrated. We find ourselves with unprecedented access to information, a sense of horizontal access to resources, and the ability to define and occupy roles that might have previously been absent from our individual existence.

Classical ashram life allows for deep immersions in the experiences and practices of *yoga*, since the residents live there full-time and do little else. Mysore style programs present an alternate method of feeling this immersion. They are characterised by quiet regularity. Students attend Mysore classes every day, or at least several times per week. The schedule is very consistent.

This style of *yoga* tends towards routine in a way that reminds us of cycles of the body and the cycles of nature. There is a great strength inherent in such a consistent approach. It becomes a part of your life and the result is a very concentrated experience. It is an efficient and practical approach that allows us to experience sagely and householder lives at the same time.

The Mysore style environment offers a way to be immersed in the energy of retreat, seclusion, relaxation, single-pointed curiosity, and earnest spiritual pursuit on a daily basis.

What is "spirituality"

The word "spirituality" means different things for many people. For some it would involve worshipping a God and following the rules of a religion.

In the context of this system of *yoga*, we treat the word "spirit" as a synonym for words like "centre", "essence", "heart", and "source". In this context, spirituality refers to the pursuit of, and identification with, the centre or essence of yourself, the primary aspect of yourself from which other levels unfold. As degraded as organised religions tend to be, most of them probably start with this sort of purpose as well.

Spirituality is a clearly definable process, spanning cultures and eras. It is a two-step, repeating cycle of concentrating deeply inwards and then relaxing expansively outwards. This pattern of action allows us to discover a profound faculty of multi-dimensional attention. In Sanskrit this central attentive point has a few names, one of which is *ātman*.

The spiritual process is an alternation between laser-like focus and wide attentiveness — intense focus on a point within, followed by broad sensitivity stretching across perceptions on the outside. The primary concern of *yoga* is the tension and play between these two aspects, leading to integration and expansion of the field of consciousness.

Spirituality is the centrepiece of poetry throughout human history. It is the primal attainment of the soul, the realisation of our platform in space. It is the perspective of reality that endures through all manner of phases and excursions. It is the gathering together of pieces to see the outlines and formation that were previously unseen. It is to access the inexhaustible pool of energy at the centre of all radiation. It is the personal witnessing of the transcendent and the immanent.

In *yoga* and spirituality, a mechanism used to elevate awareness is the uniting of polarities within one's experience. That is, to see clearly the positive and negative of each situation. To do this, empathy is invoked, and compulsive needs and aversions are resolved. This is a dissociation from extreme positions and it is known as *vairāgya.*

The active nature of this mechanism is characterised as a yoking or harnessing, using this world of apparent dualities, taking charge, and employing will and vision. This is a practised aspiration and a constant remembrance. It is called *abhyāsa*[2].

The consistent application of *abhyāsa* and *vairāgya* is the essence of *yoga*, and the combined practice is known as *sādhana*.

The mountaintop metaphor

There are many ways of describing and illustrating the spiritual dynamic, and a very useful one is the metaphor of the mountaintop and our heroic climb to the top. Our essence is the faculty of witnessing, and we sit in varying locations on a mountain. We can see everything below our location in any moment. Imagine yourself, the witnessing faculty, as a powerful searchlight. We move up and down the mountain according to our desires and reactions. The further up, the greater the area illumined by our light. The further down we go, fewer objects are included in the beam, and the greater expanses above fall dark.

Movement up the mountain is achieved by resolving polarities. Unresolved polarities keep us attached to specific places, unable to see past our attractions and aversions. Ascending the mountain is a process of surging and spiralling upwards using techniques of *yoga.* It is a cycle of earnest elevation (*abhyāsa*), followed by consolidation and expansion on a plateau (*vairāgya*), and then the cycle repeats, again and again.

Climbing the mountain improves the view of things that had seemed separate, and it is important to note that nothing is left behind, escaped, or denied. More is seen, more options and contexts, and so any previously felt need to escape falls away.

---

[2] Yoga Sutras 1.13 and 1.15

Imagine the most all-encompassing and uplifted state of mind you can. The state where everything makes sense, where you have the most wit and intelligence and creativity available. You at the top of your mountain, with the wisdom of age and the spark of youth, seeing all with clarity and poise. The "head" of yourself which is god-like, and in Sanskrit called *īśvara*[3] or *śiva,* is the faculty of "ultimate will" that exists at the top of the mountain.

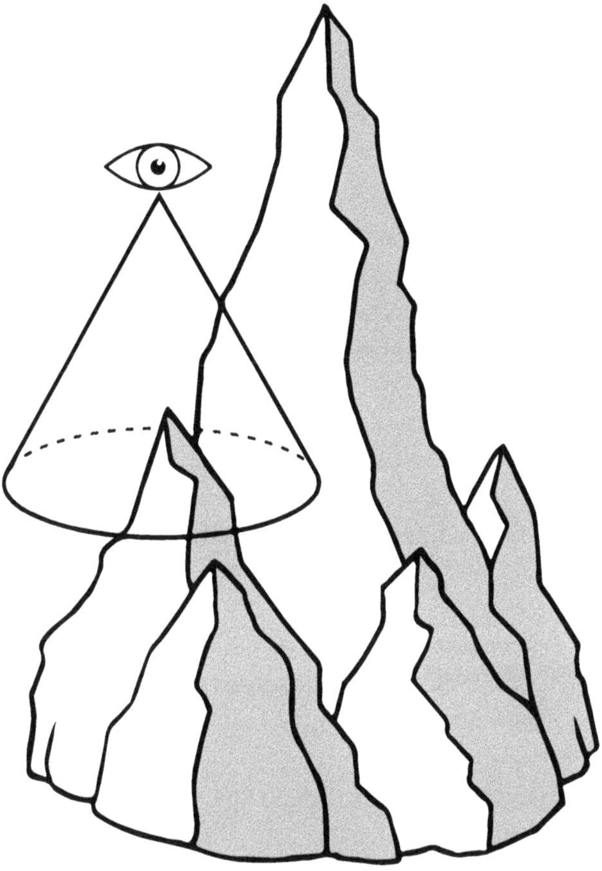

Diagram: The mountain of consciousness, its objects, and the subjective witness that moves up and down and around, with increasing and decreasing scope.

[3] Yoga Sutras 1.24

Mountaintops can be experienced as a broadening of awareness so that more of your non-conscious mind is made conscious. Eventually, there is nothing other than one integrated and fully accessible mind. The hidden or buried or forgotten parts of mind do not need to stay that way.

Those who enjoy computer science might make a comparison to the terms "data" and "information". Data refers to many separate objects which exist further down the mountain, into specificity. Information refers to a set of organised data formed coherently, this sort of object exists further up the mountain and is less easily described in words, containing many ideas and relationships. Data are facts and information is wisdom based on those facts.

The mountaintop metaphor can be elucidated through the idea of peripheral vision too. In a very practical way, it is obviously advantageous to be able to see more than one thing at a time while driving a car. The field of vision can be wide and vast when one is trained to see many things at the same time, rather than darting the gaze from one object to another.

In these examples and many more there is a realisation of greater simultaneity. The scope of awareness is increased and so is the volume of data that can be handled without feeling as though attention is splintered. In *yoga* we find a training process to go beyond previous mental limits, just as with physical training of muscles.

If it ever feels complex, pause and step back. Spirituality is very simple and is actually the default pursuit of humanity. When we are free from the artifices of sophisticated materiality, we know this to be true:

The simple practice of positive thought and action is enough.

One need only spend a little time living closer to nature to recognise this. In an isolated forest existence, your scope of awareness naturally increases, as the area surrounding you is distinctly relaxing — not filled with people and advertising messages. The air is beautiful and clean, the birds and flowers invite you to stretch outwards, the greater the stretch the more pleasure is found. This is a natural way of living, and quite at odds with city life.

Protective barriers, beyond a basic four walls, are not required. A kinship with the elements is felt, a constructive relation between you and your world takes place. All is positive in this context.

This is how to take spirituality to its zenith — the persistent and honest commitment to thoughts and actions that are both exciting to you and helpful to others, in whatever degree you are able, in each consecutive moment. This is how the mountaintop is found, in increasing measure. The witnessing faculty sees desires and beliefs weaving in amongst the reasoning intellect and idle curiosity.

When desires, intellect, and imagination are blended, *śiva* is there.

A note on modern science

Modern psychology is young, as is neuroscience. They are exciting fields that are gradually unfolding knowledge about the mind. Because these are young sciences, their findings start at the surface of truth, gradually becoming more subtle and nuanced.

Newton's laws, for example are true and accurate to an extent, and were found to break down at a certain point, and were replaced by Einstein's findings, which hold up to a greater degree. If all goes well, modern science will continue to have revelatory discoveries by visionaries that will help us find order in apparent chaos, and find determinism in apparent indeterminism.

Understand that you are a scientist as well. In fact, you are the scientist of your personal world. You decide who and what you believe, from where to draw information, how to apply logic and critical thinking. You decide the probabilities assigned to certain viewpoints, you decide if and when to ever stop questioning certain theories altogether.

If you decide to take on board the mass of knowledge given to you by your parents, teachers, and society without much scrutiny, well it is the scientist that is making that decision. The scientist is determining that all of these people and institutions appear rigorous and trustworthy enough, and that the risk of living out the entire human life with incorrect or incomplete knowledge is low enough to generally justify putting aside critical or opposing ideas. That would be a scientific conclusion that you make.

It's all a matter of degree, personally determined. You and your sense of truth, your instincts, your curiosity, your education, all play a part. It is the game of life. Played well, you may enjoy richness and fertility of the mind for one hundred years or more, played poorly you may find yourself starved of insights in a static materialism.

You are a scientist. As much as you may prefer not to be one, you are one. The buck stops with you. But we do not always trust ourselves and we do not always feel inclined to take complete responsibility for ourselves — we abdicate to experts and groups of experts.

Now, I am not saying that we should always trust every fleeting thought that occurs, I am just explaining the reason for the creation of modern scientific institutions. We are humble about our capacities and acknowledge the power of peer-review.

The academic discipline of psychology was founded in the late 19th century, for example. Neuroscience is even younger, starting in the mid-20th century. You might say that this is still a good starting point, and that it is really all we have, and it has done so much already, so why not continue? But is it all we have?

There are many household-name scientists that have much reverence for ancient Indian thought. This culture explored the mind in scientific terms for thousands of years. It is often assumed that older cultures are more primitive, but a deeper investigation reveals extraordinary scientific work being performed long ago.

Robert Oppenheimer said that the recently obtained access to texts of Indian metaphysics was one of the greatest privileges of the 20th century. He praised the Bhagavad Gītā and held the view that modern science was somewhat unwittingly refining the wisdom that had been established long ago in India[4].

Erwin Schrödinger sang the virtues of Indian thought and named the Bhagavad Gītā and Upanishads as a font of wisdom[5]. He highlighted the way they explain the paradoxical oneness and diversity that is present in our existence, the framework of a single all-encompassing consciousness that takes the temporary form of separateness.

Werner Heisenberg was working on quantum theory when he spent time as the guest of Rabindranath Tagore, who assisted Heisenberg in reconciling the seemingly crazy ideas he developing. Tagore showed him these ideas were actually the **starting point** of Indian metaphysics[6].

Nikola Tesla adopted Sanskrit terms from the Upanishads[7] to indicate his ideas on the structure of the universe and the nature of existence, saying that "all perceptible matter comes from a primary substance, or a tenuity beyond conception, filling all space, the *ākāśa* or luminiferous ether, which is acted upon by the life-giving *prāṇa* or creative force, calling into existence, in never ending cycles, all things and phenomena."

Carl Sagan famously said that while Europeans were barely starting to free themselves of the notion that the world was only a few thousand years old, the Hindus had long been thinking in cycles of billions of years[8].

---

[4] Julius Oppenheimer, *Science and the Common Understanding* (NY: Simon And Schuster, Inc., 1954)

[5] Erwin Schrödinger, *What is life?* (Cambridge: Cambridge University Press, 1944)

[6] Fritjof Capra, *Uncommon Wisdom* (New York: Simon And Schuster, Inc., 1988)

[7] Nikola Telsa, "Man's Greatest Achievement", *New York American*, 1930

[8] Carl Sagan, *Cosmos* (New York: Random House., 1988)

The science of psychology is still skimming the surface of a vastly complex thing called "mind". Neuroscience has still not discovered many connections and relationships in the brain. Physics has still not solved the mysteries that lay underneath quantum mechanics.

This is an exciting journey of discovery. As a scientist, you must acknowledge the infancy of these disciplines, and therefore take their findings as approximations, working theories, starting points. You must recall that every decade, every century, revolutions in thought take place. We get to witness the infancy of Western science.

As a scientist, you must also collect your own data and perform your own experiments. You must explore wisdom that exists outside the books found in your high school. You must also assess the groups from which you obtain information. Science used to be found in publicly-funded universities that provided free rein for visionaries to spend their lives exploring.

More recently, universities have had funding for such things slashed. There is a clear financial imperative now, a closer relationship between tertiary education and industry, an expectation of return on investment. Institutions are increasingly focused on the commercial applications of scientific discoveries.

Whereas speculative and visionary work was once lauded and economically supported by society, it is now replaced by more profitable endeavours. The study of quantum mechanics is a low status pursuit in university physics departments, viewed with a degree of suspicion. Esteemed theoretical physicist Sean Carroll shares an anecdote about writing a grant proposal and subsequently being advised to keep quiet with regard to his interests in the foundations of quantum mechanics if he wanted to be taken seriously[9]. He talks of the headstrong scientists who are frequently responsible for the significant advancements made — those willing to pursue problems that are important, if unpopular.

---

[9] Sean Carroll, *Something Deeply Hidden* (New York: Dutton, 2017)

We like to think that we are no longer the fearful mob who killed visionaries like Socrates — a philosopher executed by the State of Athens for allegedly corrupting youth with ideas that countered those of the ruling institutions, or Hypatia — a mathematician and astronomer who was dismembered by a Christian mob for the same reason. While we may not murder them, the trend is more insidious, we simply defund them. A most unscientific silence ensues.

Say that tomorrow, the science of psychology discovers that previous ideas about the brain's ability to multitask were mistaken and that the brain actually only processes one thing at a time. How would this affect your cognition if you were to believe it to be true? You could buy in to that belief system and work within those agreed upon limits.

But is this wise? Modern science makes findings using the current level of knowledge and the accuracy of current technology. It might change again in a few years. Is it a good idea to force the peg of your understanding to fit the hole of current theories?

Conversely, you could believe that you have a searchlight of attention that moves up and down and around a mountain made of objects. Those objects are within consciousness and are of varying subtlety. You can effortlessly position your searchlight to illuminate objects to suit your desires and requirements, and you can instantly see anything you need. You can zoom in to see something specific very clearly, or zoom out to see the operation of a system with all of its parts moving in elaborate patterns.

This is the claim made by ancient Indian scientists. They found it is replicable and they give instructions for you, the scientist, to experience the results of the experiment. Will you close your eyes to that and prefer the option provided by a much younger tradition of inquiry?

Form your own probability matrix

A true scientist is one who develops their own mind, their higher faculties, their memory, and their capacity for abstract thought. Rather than acquiescing when told they are "limited", a true scientist sees this as a call to action.

There is no need to completely hand over the search for truth to others. We all have the capacity to pursue greater understanding and deeper perception. It could even be said that this is a moral duty, a *dharma*.

Yes, it's well known that humans engage in wishful thinking, and that many examples exist of people suspending their credulity and following charismatic leaders down a problematic path. But that ought not to dim our search for insight, instead it should indicate the need for collaboration and peer-review, and funding!

Scientists consider hypotheses and perform experiments. It is unscientific to refuse to experiment simply because the potential conclusions are uncomfortable. To do that would be to yield to fear. In fact, a culture that blends fear and materialism can lead to a nihilism or fatalism that is utterly disempowering and opens one up for the very exploitation we seek to avoid.

Science is morality

Psychology informs us that our brains are unreliable, that our memories are reconstructed and littered with bias. We have been told that a simple stroll down the street involves having our visual field consist of a few directly observed objects while the rest is assumed and filled in based on prior experience.

On this point, ancient Indian thought agrees. There is much agreement actually. The Indian repository of knowledge just tends to have additional useful information along with the superficial empirical findings of psychology and neurology.

See, all memory is constructed. Not just long-term memory — everything. What happened a few minutes ago, the previous paragraph, your plans for tomorrow, your daydreams and night dreams. All exist on the same level. They are all equally real. They are all projections in your consciousness, filtered by your beliefs, emotions, thoughts.

You are constructing everything in the present moment. Looking at someone standing in front of you, remembering your last holiday, imagining next Christmas — all have the same value. All that exists does so in the present moment.

One must be comfortable with this

Discomfort with this idea leads to coping mechanisms such as recording history, storing and documenting things, planning and investments, accumulation and hoarding. These are ways to soothe us and create a sense of permanence outside the present moment. But the past and future are identical in their nature — they exist in imagination alone.

The amount of attention you pay to the present moment matters a great deal. Watch your beliefs, emotions, thoughts, and actions dance upon the screen of your reality.

This is all too much sometimes, especially if you have grown up with a sense of there being certain things that are concrete. But their concreteness is a convenience, a relic from the days of classical physics. You can maintain that, or something else. It is up to you, the scientist.

The cultural consequence of needing certainty is the mistaken belief that the totality of existence consists of that which is visible or known. We begin to solely identify with the most obvious aspects of the brain: the elements that arise from mammalian biology. This has a self-fulfilling effect. We focus on phenomena and symptoms that are easily viewed, and we tend to forget about our higher functions.

A group hypnosis occurs where everyone agrees that their brains are inherently unreliable because science has "proven it", and therefore we need to be told what is true rather than pursue the truth ourselves. We start to forget about our own genius, and the geniuses of our history. We become so blind to the extraordinary that we define gifted children as having disorders.

Pursue your highest purpose

It's very important to back yourself. We have very capable intellects. You are able to modify your own mind and to be explorative. You are not a victim of the world — you are the author of it. In this practice of *yoga*, not only do we want to personally feel as content and potent as possible, we also want to have a clear vision for how we apply this state of mind in a purposeful way in the world.

We want to go beyond being caught up in personal pleasure, beyond the intoxication of our own enjoyment. As we become richer, with greater technology, our ability to destroy or improve the world increases. We can go up just as fast as we can go down, and what determines the direction is our will and our beliefs.

Do you personally believe that you can vastly improve the world? If this belief is not present, ask yourself why, and who gave you the counter-view. Check where your beliefs are drawn from, and who benefits from you subscribing to those views. Everything you experience is translated by your senses, habits, and assumptions. In *yoga*, this is referred to as the *koṣa*-s, layers or sheathes of progressively subtle assumptions. Indeed, neuroscience presents the brain as a filter which performs "sensory gating", filtering vast inputs into something very specific.

You can modify these filters according to your will and preferences, all the things that interest or excite you. It is a good idea to investigate the extent to which you believe you can change yourself, and how much effect you believe it will have on the world. You have complete agency and potency, and it is astonishing what one person can achieve in this domain.

So much of our mind is dedicated to the task of looking, seeking, checking, identifying. We are carrying the tendencies of mammals to be hyper-vigilant towards danger. The creatures who donated much of our DNA survived because they were able to spot the tiny little signs of danger, a set of eyes peering from within the bushes. But, while paranoia is a virtue in the jungle, it is not so helpful now. The wiring is still there, waiting for something to run from, something to attack. But it does not need to be activated in this way, and the way triggers are pressed into service is completely under our control.

In *yoga*, that incessant vigilance to spot danger is used in service of higher and more adaptive ideals. One may habituate the noticing of opportunities to creatively express positivity. In doing so, the intention to live as scientific and creative explorers on a journey of understanding is consciously impressed upon the circuitry.

Tools are used to form new habits. This is why affirmations and rituals are frequently seen in spiritual and psychological systems of wellbeing. Many options are available, and we will explore some of them later.

So, be hungry for inspiration.

Be part of a community that will hold you to account.

2

MYSORE STYLE IS FOR BEGINNERS

It is really only suitable for beginners

The students who have the easiest introduction to Mysore style classes are often those who have no notion of what to expect in a class. They might have read about *yoga*, or their doctor or friends suggested it.

Unaware of different styles of *yoga* class, they just arrive and place themselves in the class to be taught how to practice. They experience a gradual and healthy unfoldment of physical ability and comfort, developing quickly into feelings of expansion and joy.

At the start, a Mysore style teacher will assume that you know nothing at all about *yoga* and walk you through the fundamentals. All of these are covered: the basics of the practice, what sort of attitude and expectations to cultivate, the way to breathe, how to monitor your energy, and of course the physical postures.

So begins the process of being taught each shape, one-at-a-time, with the teacher paying attention to your skeletal structure, your current abilities and limitations, your imbalances and endurance. At the same time, you also enter into dialogue with the teacher; you let them know about areas of pain or uncertainty.

In the first few months you will have relatively more dialogue with the teacher than those who have been practicing for a while. This is very natural and logical. It is a mixed-levels class, so there will be all levels of students present as well as you, doing all manner of interesting things. Enjoy being inspired by their presence. Everyone all together, people of all ages and experience levels, sharing a common interest.

Moments of vulnerability

Whatever your level of experience, you will have moments of vulnerability and feeling like a beginner; that is guaranteed. Sometimes you'll find yourself standing there with no idea what comes next. You can assign to that experience a positive meaning. Treat this as a moment to rest, relax, maybe look around the room.

You will notice that most people need a hand from time to time to remember or to have something explained. When you find yourself unsure what to do next, and the teacher is speaking to someone else, just wait and they will soon come to you and teach you how to do the next pose or answer your question.

Within a few months you'll be doing things that you were previously certain you could not possibly do. You may even have the sweet experience of noticing a brand new first-timer enter the room and appear as overwhelmed as you once did. Even after a few years of practice you will still need to sometimes pause and ask for help. Again and again, this experience of relying on a friendly resource continues until you are an expert and have achieved perfection in every sense — which never actually occurs of course!

This process trains us to be comfortable within ourselves, knowing we are allowed to be vulnerable. So, embrace the relief of being a beginner in some sense, the experience of life opening new doors that contain new adventures and things to learn, of being free to flop around carefree as a child, and have space held for you.

Working through trepidation and insecurity brings an enormous amount of growth in itself. It is common to experience feelings of not being adequately smart or strong or flexible. Often people will ponder if they should study at home first before entering the school, which is of course a backwards approach. All that is needed to practice in Mysore style classes is a desire to learn, and your regular attendance.

It is ironic that complete beginners, who don't know anything about styles of *yoga*, waltz into the studio and have a great time learning poses and having experiences of progression, while experienced participants and even instructors of led classes often feel intimidated by the idea of being taught in the Mysore style. Each individual would explain their resistance in their own terms, but it could be perhaps generalised as feelings of self-consciousness, feeling lost and embarrassed, as though they should somehow know more about something they have never experienced — these feelings seem to prevail.

The public image of Ashtanga Vinyasa Yoga highlights the elite level practitioners who perform amazing feats of strength and contortion — but who make up only a moderate proportion of total students world-wide. The class is actually set up for complete beginners. What a shame it would be for people to think they need to qualify or perform in order to attend.

The best thing Mysore style teachers can do is to encourage experienced students to embrace feeling new to *yoga* again, to step out of the expert persona, and relax into a wide-eyed beginner state. It is quite an indulgence to be able to flop around on the mat, feel experimental, and learn new things.

Here is a testimony from a new student who already had experience with led classes, and had even completed a modern Teacher Training course.

> *"I remember the first time walking into the studio and realising that I had a very long way to go. I decided to take the mindset of a complete beginner and act as though I was learning from scratch. Seeing others around me so dedicated to the practice motivated me to continually come back. Once I learnt the sequence, the practice became much more than just physically strengthening and lengthening the muscles. It became a beautiful opportunity to focus on my breath and sink into a relaxed, meditative state."*

Let's provide a safe space for all. If it helps, we can encourage instructors of led classes to just come and do their own sequences. After all, the space is there to be shared. The intention and purpose of *yoga* is to help all comers have a more enjoyable life, not to insist upon a specific dogma. This means accommodating the emotional and physical needs of people — modifying our approach from the idealised template.

When I discovered Mysore style

With all of that said, I personally did not have a nervous first-time experience of Mysore style. I found the class as a result of the convergence of a few events: my girlfriend broke up with me all of a sudden, a few days after Christmas. Additionally, the led *yoga* studio I had been attending for the last nine months — where I had been practicing for the first time since high school — had closed down for an entire month to replace their floor.

Shocked and heartbroken from the relationship break-up, I found myself wanting to cry if I sat down at home, so I would ride my bicycle aimlessly for hours and hours a day. It was the Christmas holidays and I had loads of time on my hands, time that was now utterly empty.

During the night I would wake in physical pain. Excessive bicycling and a sudden cessation of my stretching routine resulted in very tight legs. In desperation I did a web search for "Yoga Newcastle". I knew nothing of *yoga* styles and the first result that came up was Ashtanga Yoga Newcastle, so I gave them a call. I explained that I needed an alternate studio for a few weeks and expressed concern that the style of class at the studio might not be strong enough for me. I recall the wry, knowing tone of her response: they would definitely be able to provide a sufficiently challenging practice for me.

I fully expected to "wow" them. I remember walking in that first time and immediately having that expectation removed! I saw middle-aged men and women putting their legs behind the head and floating through the air on their hands. So began a wonderful period for me.

The timing was perfect in many ways as you can see due to those circumstances, but also due to a plateau I had begun to feel. I had a fair degree of fitness and had attacked those powerful and heated led *yoga* classes for almost a year — and I mean attacked — I did nine classes per week every week! This was in alongside a corporate career involving 70 hours a week of work and driving. Maybe that's a contributing factor to my girlfriend breaking up with me...

I know exactly what would have happened if I had continued with those led classes. In the early stages of my practice, the sheer difficulty of doing the fundamental poses had forced me to develop inward concentration and this resulted in a quieting of the mind. But I had already started to notice that the need to be focused was reducing. I could now do the poses and there was again space for idle inner chatter.

If I had stuck with led classes, I would have continued to experience a reduction of consciousness-based benefits and I would have sought to find them again by becoming more extreme, or grasping for poses to entertain me, eventually getting bored and possibly moving on to something else, having completely missed the point of *yoga*.

Mysore style gave me a direct experience of pure attention by means of a repetitive series of postures, practiced quietly in a group of friendly people, under the close supervision of a very experienced teacher.

Previously, in led classes, I would occasionally experience deep revelatory experiences, here and there — most often in the *śavāsana* part at the end of class. But with Mysore style those experiences occur frequently during each practice. It becomes quite easy to get out of bed early in the morning when such a gift awaits.

Let us have a life-long practice

The Mysore style framework offers a life-long and sustainable practice, a loving and caring space with expert teachers and supportive fellow students learning, collectively and individually, about their capacities and tendencies.

Any *yoga* postures can be practiced in a Mysore style environment, and the series of postures most commonly practiced belong to the well-known Ashtanga Vinyasa Yoga system. Most modern led classes are also based on this particular system, with its posture sequences, consisting of increasingly challenging movements.

Ashtanga Vinyasa Yoga practiced in a Mysore style setting represents a life-long and complete approach to *yoga* for all people. The series of postures ought to be seen as a loose framework for play and experimentation over the entire lifespan.

An ideal teacher will help students jump around like a monkey when they are young and brimming with excess energy and loads of resilience. They will also help people manage changes in the body as they mature, helping balance solar and lunar attributes over time, that is, *yang* and *yin*[10].

---

[10] The commercial imperative to fit as many customers as possible into a class is what has driven the prevalence of led classes. It is an experiment in a large-scale, one-size-fits-all delivery of *yoga*. In recent years, we have seen a somewhat lumbering approach

In *yoga*, we aim is to proactively reveal issues that lie under the surface, issues that will probably arise at some point in our lives. The idea is to discover them sooner, in the safe and controlled space of the classroom, so that they can be transformed and harnessed consciously. In this way, lessons can be learned far more effectively and there is a reduced likelihood of them sprouting at inopportune times in our lives.

The solar, or *yang*, tendency manifests in adherence to systems with excessive strictness or zealotry, potentially resulting in injury or even aggressive behaviour. The lunar, or *yin*, tendency can manifest as passivity or a free-form, do-as-you-feel approach that skips over the true needs of the student, resulting in lack of progress, boredom, or resignation.

A complete practice is designed to reveal such aspects and provide the perfect space to resolve them. When difficulties arise during practice, the teacher and student work together to diagnose and rehabilitate with the approach of a sort of hybrid jungle-doctor-physiotherapist. This empowered collaboration enriches the student with education about human anatomy and their own ability to heal and enhance themselves.

The practice is continually adapted to suit how the student is feeling and what the body is signalling. The light of consciousness is directed to any aspect that raises its hand through pain, discomfort, or incapacity. Such signals are respectfully acknowledged and a dialogue is established.

In a Mysore style setting with an expert teacher and a healthy collaborative dialogue, students can have deep inner experiences and notice their hidden needs. At every opportunity the teacher reminds the students:

You are here to learn about yourself, to understand how to manage goals and setbacks from a physical and emotional stance.

---

to balancing classes. Softer and more restorative classes have emerged where passive stretching is practiced, without the usual dynamic and heating transitions. Combination *yin/yang* classes are additionally offered to simulate the balance that is already immediately available in Mysore style classes.

Change is the only constant

In Mysore style *yoga* there is moment-to-moment dynamism involving *yin* and *yang* and all the gradations in between. Different teachers have wildly varying views on how the guidelines of the Ashtanga Vinyasa system ought to be applied, how strictly, how much creative modification should occur, and under what circumstances. Certainly, in the past, a blinkered and authoritarian approach has been easy to find.

Generally, a hard-line or strict teacher matures, and if they persist in this field for ten years or more, they come to see the value in modifying practices. The traditions are allowed to be less of a focal point, supplanted by insight into how to improve lives through the process of *yoga*, allowing them to have a life-long practice.

When a student has a strong imbalance or other postural need, it can be necessary to make a departure from the normal progression of poses. A common example is seen in students with forward set shoulders, tending towards kyphosis. Often such a student will benefit vastly from the early introduction of back-bending postures that involve drawing the shoulders back, strengthening rhomboids etc. In this case, the teacher must be willing to prescribe postures that a traditionalist might not allow.

If a teacher is unwilling to go in a therapeutic direction, it can be harmful to the student. Steadfastly requiring the student to perform according to a tradition can negatively affect their posture and their life.

A key intention of *yoga* must be remembered:

***Yoga* is about experiencing — and helping others experience — states of happiness, clarity, and authorship more frequently.**

Enthusiasm ought to be harnessed

A fallacy of spiritual culture is that in striving for balance one must arrive at a bland passivity. This is an incomplete view. The practice is to locate edges and limitations in the body and the mind. To find middle ground by actively seeking the extremes — to see them clearly so that in each moment one's position can be adjusted to suit.

It is practiced in these terms: go wild when you want to, relax and regroup when you want to. Eventually expand and elevate and find yourself to be viewing a scene of clarity and potential action that is broad and safe and exciting. Harness enthusiasm and identify predispositions toward conservatism or rebellion. It is desirable to have access to both modes of behaviour.

For many, it is most natural to spend the initial years of practice being a strict adherent. During this time, one is held to a standard beyond what is immediately attainable. Much is learned here — the rules of the system and a great deal of inner strength. Then, after a few years it can be appropriate to start breaking the rules and noticing the benefit in alternative versions of postures, in changing or adding things.

An even greater strength is attained here as students recognise their ability to be their own teacher — having first "earned it". Practice enters a new phase of exploration that is safe due to the grounding of the previous.

You are the author

This is a demonstration of the ultimate skill: to see the totality of every situation and then create with greater effectiveness. Every situation is a blank slate waiting for an individual to give it a meaning. In all cases, it is the individual who decides, and these decisions can be conscious, or they can be unconscious.

To defer to an external authority or social consensus for a value judgement is a valid choice, but even so, it is a choice. You, the individual, assigns the eventual meaning. You are the final authority.

There is a cultural habit of viewing the world as an array of things wanted and things unwanted. It can be hard to see the neutrality in things — the normal operation is to reflexively give things meaning based on habit or assumption without conscious consideration, thus moving mechanically along a path of ups and downs, largely unaware of the ability to pause, see the flip-side and make a new selection.

> *"Thoughts of both virtue and error are creations of the intellect. Consciousness exposes those creations entwined in their domain[11]."*

The spiritual practice is one of understanding this concept and implementing the vision in our lives, to see the neutrality of every event and to then select a positive meaning according to your own preference. You are the agent who assigns meaning to events. You are the ultimate controller of your subjective experience.

The only thing that we truly know to be existent is our personal subjective consciousness. The "outside world" is a theoretical concept that exists in your mind. This is not controversial in a scientific sense, even though it may be unsettling. When you perceive a person talking to you, you are watching a show in your mind. We are essentially hallucinating our perceived reality. Everything is a dream. Everything occurs in your imagination.

[11] Śaṅkara, *Laghu Vākya Vṛtti, śloka 7*

The totality of existence is the faculty of consciousness, and all objects are displayed upon it.

You may act as though the objective world exists outside of you, but as a scientist, you have to concede this is an assumption. All perception plays as an image in your mind. No matter how external it "seems", or how objective it "feels", or how many apparently existing human beings agree with us — the scientist in us must concede that we have chosen to operate on the assumption that it is real. This is the postulate of Western materialism — that there is an outside world separate to consciousness. We tend to gloss over the fact that this is a quietly declared assumption.

Materialists use their consciousness to adopt the views of materialism. They use their consciousness to decide that objects they perceive in their own consciousness exist outside of their consciousness. This is a logical short circuit that results in confused definitions and unsolvable puzzles. Furthermore, they use their consciousness, which is the totality of their existence, to diminish consciousness itself to an emergent quirk of nature. They use their unlimited power to declare themselves limited.

Having established a dissonant but stable baseline, scientific culture then experiments within its self-imposed limits. Theories are tested, evidence is collected — all by means of consciousness — using objects that have been assumed to be real. Evidence is reviewed by figments of our mind who we call "peers," who we also pretend are real.

The only thing that is empirically real, however, is "I".

This sort of discussion is not valued much in our current scientific culture. Instead, there is a general agreement to proceed as though the objective world exists as something separate from us, and that we exist inside it, and that consciousness is an emergent property of biology.

Yoga acknowledges that you are the ultimate arbiter of reality. It begins with the universal empirical truth that all is in consciousness.

Actively attend to the upside

A positive, negative, or neutral meaning can be ascribed to all things.

Frequently it is observed that inspirational and successful people had adversity in their lives that compelled them to develop great inner resources. The ability to lift oneself up and create positive situations is a well-known counterbalance to difficulty in life. Knowing it is possible to identify the positive meaning in all things that you experience, it stands as the most logical path to take, as much as we are able.

If enjoyment is desired, then we ought to take the time to identify the enjoyable aspects of all situations. This is self-evident. In situations that seem negative, positivity ought to be sought, and in situations that already seem positive, further positivity ought to be sought. To deliberately identify and assign a positive meaning to absolutely everything is the attitude that results in an ecstatic and creative life.

Humans being habitual creatures, the tendency is to behave along automatic paths, encountering and reacting to stimuli in a mechanical fashion. In *bhakti yoga* the practice is of using the will to pause, elevate, search, and select paths of action with conscious awareness. It is to recognise the newness of each moment. The term *bhakti* means dedication to the higher perspective. Sometimes this term evokes more modern religious notions, but it is not necessary.

When practicing *bhakti yoga*, one is devoted to the project of enhancing vision and intent. When one performs the work of persistently making this decision, attentively administering the approach to each moment, there is a sacrifice of inertia into the furnace of aspiration. Flame on!

Attention is service

The primary function of consciousness is attention, and to attend to something is to serve it. It is what you are born to do. It is what you are always doing. You are freely giving all of your attention to something at all times. It's so easy and pleasurable to give attention to someone, to serve them, when you feel a certain affection toward them. Sometimes, you get to unleash it upon another human, sometimes you give it to a hobby, and other times you give it to social media feeds and traffic jams.

The beginning and middle and end of every one of your actions is contained within your consciousness. There is nothing you can perceive that is not within your consciousness. The totality of you is consciousness. Nothing is known except this.

When you pay attention to an object, you are using your consciousness to attend to a figure within your consciousness. When you serve someone, you are serving a figure within your consciousness. It is obvious that all of your actions ought to be positive and integrative, since they are actions directed from yourself to yourself. Love directed to another is love directed to yourself. This is not a romantic platitude; it is mechanical and literal. Sometimes figures in your consciousness *seem* to move according to a force or will from outside yourself, but this is a surface appearance, and a scientist searches for the truth beneath appearances.

There is an enigmatic Sanskrit statement that "the effects of devotion are of an identical form"[12]. This indicates a duplication or reciprocation of efforts, rather than a hard-earned production. This reflects the difference between mindsets of scarcity and abundance. The fruits of devotion are duplicated and the universe expands to make room for them. There is no sense of taking devotion from one person in order to give it to yourself. There is an infinite supply.

---

[12] Narada Bhakti Sutras *śloka* 30

Aspiration results in yet more aspiration. The exertion and effort that characterises the start of the process of elevating your perspective are temporary. A threshold is eventually crossed as the new habit is formed and you see positive aspects clearly without struggle. This effortlessness is a result of the harmonisation of parts of the being that had formerly been categorised, segregated, and treated as separate. It consumes energy, keeping things apart and maintaining separation.

Take, for example, the difference between a devotional and a scientific attitude. Devotional attitudes reflect a desire for empathy, to feel the feelings of another, which is knowledge by direct perception. Likewise, the intellectual scientific search is dedicated to knowledge — only this time it occurs by the act of measurement.

The difference between devotion and science is one of technique rather than principle. The principle is the same, the motive is the same, and the investment of sincerity and enthusiasm is the same. People may invest effort in arguing this point for a while, but anyone who wishes to grow must put aside pontificating and bickering, and allow all aspects of the human being to work together to bring about the ultimate outcome of transcendental knowledge.

Ultimately, there really is only one energy — and it is embracing, enthusiastic, seeking, permissive, constructive, and all-encompassing.

No longer does emotion need to be viewed with distrust by the intellect, and no longer does intellect need to be shunned by the artist. No longer held apart in water-tight compartments, the highest pursuit of humanity is the complete and harmonious action of former halves, becoming one.

Perception of bodily sensations

Consider the way that sensation in the physical body is perceived. The sensation of tightness can be positively experienced as excitement.

Often this occurs quite naturally, tightness is simply stored-up pleasure, accompanied by anticipation of glorious release. Tightness is often experienced first as a negative, as pain, and then as joy as it is transformed. When there is an automatic understanding that tightness is freedom, waiting to be unlocked, it ceases to be a cause of distress.

Mental forms of tightness, like nervousness and apprehension, can transform into thrill and delight. The anticipation of things like first-kisses, public speaking, and sky-diving builds up and is usually released as a very positive experience. The more you look for this dynamic, the more you will see it and be able to use it. When this fundamental knowledge is present, we adapt very quickly. No longer do we need to avoid discomfort. In fact, we can wholly accept it and see the upside.

Once we know the mechanism, once we understand that fear and tightness is the wrapping paper and that a joyous gift lies within, then the entirety of our experience can be enjoyed! Not just parts that are labelled as "good".

Remember that while we may act as though we **are** our bodies, they are really just another object that we perceive on the field of consciousness. Everything appears in your consciousness. You operate a body and it is within you. *Yoga* regards this contemplation as fundamental, and enthusiastic exploration yields a lifetime of benefit.

Your sensory experiences are all a construction in your imagination — an interplay of content. On the surface, it seems like there are many outside objects affecting your body, and it may be the case, but that would be an assumption, beyond what is known to be true. What is known is that you are consciousness, and pieces of content are interacting within you.

In the West, recent research into the nature of physical pain is provoking similar contemplation. On the surface, pain seems relatively simple: injury to the body causes pain, and pain reflects the state of health of the body. However, it has been discovered that much of the experience of pain is not related to the state of the tissues. In fact, the longer the pain has existed, the less related it is to the actual health of the tissues. Pain is frequently a remnant of a long-gone incident that caused psychological and physiological distress. The relationship between objects in consciousness is more malleable than previously assumed.

Consider also the notion of *interoception*, a phrase coined in the early 20th century meaning **the detection and perception of sensations in the body** including the organs and muscles. It is sensory perception — the same kind that we use to detect objects on the outside of our bodies — but directed **within** our bodies. People can perceive sensations in parts of their body such as heart-rate, movements in the intestines, even subtleties in reproductive system flows.

There is growing evidence showing that interoception plays an important role in a healthy mental existence. The attitudes and feelings people have about their body appears contingent on interoceptive ability[13]. Major depression and poor decision-making ability are linked to deficits in interoception[14]. Accurate and balanced perception of internal bodily signals seems to improve emotional regulation and awareness, and therefore reduces stress[15].

---

[13] Badoud and Tsakirisac, "From the body's viscera to the body's image: Is there a link between interoception and body image concerns?" Neuroscience & Biobehavioral Reviews, Vol. 77, June 2017

[14] Furman et al., "Interoceptive awareness, positive affect, and decision making in Major Depressive Disorder," Journal of Affective Disorders, Vol. 151, Issue 2, November 2013

[15] Price, Hooven, "Interoceptive Awareness Skills for Emotion Regulation: Theory and Approach of Mindful Awareness in Body-Oriented Therapy (MABT)," Frontiers in Psychology, May 28 2018

The importance of subtle perceptions, and the indistinct relationship between sensations and what we call physical objects, surely motivates the curious scientist to inquire deeper than superficial and sense-based effects. The obvious next step here is to wonder what an enhancement of bodily and emotional awareness could deliver in terms of accelerated human flourishing. This is an idea that is acknowledged and yet under-researched[16].

Thankfully we can research it ourselves, on ourselves. On this note, there is a lovely quirk in the naming of the old *yoga* hall in the suburb of Gokulam, Mysore. It is called the Ashtanga Yoga Research Institute. Rather than being called a studio, it is a place of research and study.

In Mysore style we develop vast interoception

In Mysore style classes, the teacher teaches you how to do each pose in a way that accommodates your body type, skeletal variations, and so forth. Then, crucially, you are directed to do the pose yourself, completely independently rather than at the same time as everyone else in the room. Each at their own pace. You are directed to practice the posture and notice the inner sensations as they change during the course of a long inhale, and then a long exhale, and then more inhales and exhales. You then do the pose again tomorrow, and every day.

This is very much like the concept of *kata* in karate; patterns of movements, carried out with precision and attention to breath and body. The movements are practiced by the student at their own pace, with guidance and correction from the teacher. This is unlike a Western style led class and it is how students can both refine their physical technique and reach deeper states of concentrative awareness more easily.

---

[16] Murphy et al., "Interoception and psychopathology: A developmental neuroscience perspective," Developmental Cognitive Neuroscience, Vol. 23, February 2017

The practice of a consist set of poses reveals the extraordinary variety of inner sensations available — the rich array of information, tactile feedback, and sensuous experiences beneath the skin. The regularity of practice creates a canvas to notice increasingly subtle changes, and a landscape upon which sensitivity blossoms, with calm and clarity.

Interoception is not developed very effectively in a group fitness style of *yoga* class, where the attention of students is reaching out to the voice of an instructor, often with accompanying music. In the same way, when a student does not know which pose is coming up next, or is distracted by excessive artificial heat, it is not possible to focus deeply on the internal.

The *yogin*-s of the Indus Valley were tuned in to this thousands of years ago and interoception has, in fact, been thoroughly researched and practiced. They determined that sensitivity can be increased over the entire duration of the physical life, and when done gradually using techniques that permit an increasing capacity to handle such sensitivity, the result is spectacular. A sense of "vision" emerges that is so extraordinary as to provoke attempts at description that are poetic and mystical. Nonetheless, it is real, and it is the natural outcome of evolution, to be enjoyed to the extent that you personally choose.

Here is an exercise to help you play with your capacity for awareness of relative electrical activation over the terrain of your available nerve and neural circuitry:

For a moment, activate your left quadriceps muscle to the exclusion of other parts of the body. Develop this local awareness. To do so you will need to be able to narrow your focus onto a very specific set of nerves in your body. Once you can do this, develop the ability to activate it without any accessory muscles switching on. Do not allow the hamstrings or adductors to activate.

Notice the limits of ability in really focusing electrical activity on a specific part of the body. Notice also your ability to reduce competing brain functions, like twitching in the torso, instability in the breath, or the subtle expression of frustration.

As the scope of this task is expanded, one will readily go beyond coarse musculature and into subtle aspects of perception and mentality. A fine-grained dexterity is cultivated in the body-mind system.

Here are some more examples:

- Notice the feeling of your ribs opening and closing as you breathe deeply. Notice the regions in your torso where this sensation is vivid and those where there is not much sensation.
- Notice the difference in sensation when your lungs are 70% full as compared to 80% full. Feel the skin gliding over bones as you breathe, notice the extent to which it feels like an upwards or sideways movement.
- Notice that when you **decide** to reach across your desk to pick something up — before you move your arm at all, your intrinsic core stabiliser muscles switch on, increasing intra-abdominal pressure and tensing the thoracolumbar fascia in preparation for the intended reaching and lifting[17].
- Pay attention to the fine mental movements that occur when you are trying to remember something, particularly when it's on the tip of your tongue and just out of reach.
- Witness the current proportion of content in your mind of an emotional nature and that of an analytical nature.
- Survey the co-existence of silent inner dialogue and associated concepts and memories that bounce around your consciousness.

---

[17] As is known to be the case — postural reflexes activate in advance of anticipated movement or balance correction needs. Hodges et al., "Three dimensional preparatory trunk motion precedes asymmetrical upper limb movement," Gait & Posture, Vol. 11, Issue 2, April 2000

"One year of Mysore style" – a testimony

"Imagine you have a car, a really fancy, ultra-modern, futuristic one. It has all these crazy features. It took FOREVER to develop as a product and it can do some really incredible things. You're stoked to have it, if somewhat baffled by it. You're not sure how it really works. You can sit in the driver's seat and press the button that turns on the engine.

You know how to move the gearstick, how to accelerate and how to brake. It's got a lot of fancy buttons and displays inside, but you don't know what they do and you're scared you will break the car if you start messing with them. You heard that there are many cool and different things that people can do with their cars, but you have no idea how. You should be able to drive it through a river and up a mountain, but you just hang out in the same places a lot because you're scared to drive the car very far away.

You should be able to drive really fast, or really slow, or through a scenic route. But you can't. Worse, there's a pretty shit radio station stuck on the stereo and you don't know how to turn it off.

This is an analogy for being in the body. We do yoga because it teaches us how to change gears, drive through rivers and across mountains. It teaches us how to stop and go, slow down and speed up, how to maximise efficiency. We learn how to clean, refuel, perform maintenance, how to delicately manoeuvre the vehicle. Gradually we learn how to change the radio station or turn it off.

The body is your main tool while you are here in this lifetime – you can and should learn how to use it to the full extent of its abilities. Mysore style has taught me this."
– Mysore student.

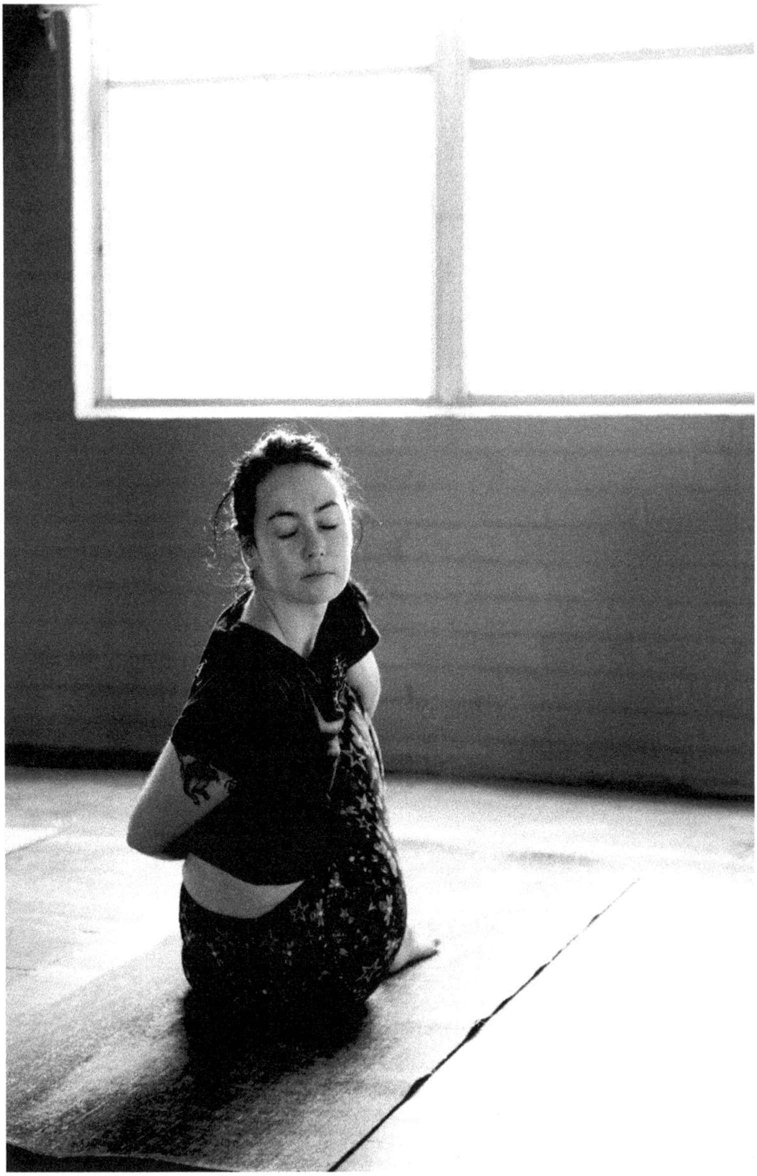

Photo credit: Kate Binnie

3

HOW TO PRACTICE

Always remember the main intention

At all points of the *yoga* journey, it is crucial to remember that our overarching intention is help ourselves and others to directly experience states of happiness and clarity more frequently and completely.

Reasons, techniques, and descriptions vary, but there is a universal claim made by all styles of *yoga* that there is a blissful existence that is available to all. The purpose of the practice is to increase the number and duration of enlightened, intuitive, and peaceful states. The physical practices of *yoga* are key to this. The postures, called *āsana*, can support this by putting more energy in the system while also increasing one's capacity for the very same energy.

For any kind of practice to support positive outcomes, it must be both challenging and safe. Increased energy without sufficient capacity results in anxiety and tension. Increased capacity without sufficient energy results in torpidity. A dynamic balance must be struck. In the realm of *yoga* postures, this means avoiding situations of both monotonous and unthinking drudgery on the one hand, and an amped-up approach where you are always trying to do tricks, on the other hand.

A Mysore style class ensures this balance is maintained on a day-to-day basis, with bespoke sequences of movement and breath, accompanied by eagle-eyed supervision, corrections and enhancements, from mature and loving teachers.

Know the ancient roots

There is a Sanskrit term, *sanātan dharma*, which means "enduring purpose", and it pre-dates Western ideas of religion and science. Regarded as the originating principle of all other Indian schools, including *yoga*, it refers to the understanding of life, the sum of knowledge and ways of being that existed in India long before colonisation.

There was a time — perhaps a mythic one — in humanity's childhood when all people were highly spiritual and far less materially oriented. The purpose for life was centred around experiential flourishing of the individual and community in a way that reflected joy and peace and aspiration. It was easy to remain centred as the all-encompassing Self called *śiva* at the top of the mountain, witnessing distinct material forms below, viewing all as ephemera within consciousness. The knowledge was ever-present, having never been forgotten.

These people had direct, continuous, and obvious awareness that they were much bigger than their physical body. They could tell that they existed for many metres beyond their body, that they were superimposed over the reality that they witness with the senses. It was a natural fact of life that their feelings, tones, and thoughts radiated outwards and were apprehended by others. Similarly, they knew that feelings they personally apprehended were frequently from others.

For these people, it was not a matter of conjecture, they could see it as clearly as we see any object. It was not philosophy — it was direct perception of reality, as clear and true as we consider our sense perceptions to be. In such a state of awareness, ethics does not really exist. Everyone enjoys positive experience, everyone accepts positive feelings from others, and everyone cultivates positivity for themselves and others.

Consciousness is a field, in Sanskrit called *puruṣa*. It is possible to identify the one whole field, which is commonly called the universe. More often, we identify with fields of a narrower scope, and we call those fields individual entities or persons within the whole. The *puruṣa* is the unchanging field of awareness on which things play out, it is the "I am". It is the light that has always been switched on and has never been switched off. It has lit up everything that has ever occurred in your experience. It is fundamentally invulnerable to distraction, it is not addicted to any activities whatsoever, so can be a perfect witness[18].

In this state of awareness, ethics is so obvious that there does not need to even be a word for it. Similarly, religious organisations have no purpose. In this state there really is no stress either. If a proximal arrangement is unpleasant, one can simply move their body and their field away from one situation and toward another.

The story goes that as people continued to create and interact with material forms, over time a forgetfulness accumulated. Now, forgetting is a consciously employed trick that humans use frequently. It allows us to re-experience or re-learn. Sometimes we deliberately forget in order to have an experience of "the first time" again. For example, we might go deliberately without a favourite food, television program, or person, for a while so that when we do again indulge, we have a fresh joy of remembering how good it feels. This is the direction that humanity travelled along — having the gift of total awareness, and choosing to forget it for the joy of remembering.

For example, we know that physical bodies and objects are coalesced energy, they are arrangements of patterns of a fluid magnetic and electrical energy. This is not controversial. The convention of labelling objects as solid and separate is a convenience, a throwback to classical physics that was superseded 100 years ago.

---

[18] Yoga Sutras 1.16

Atomic structures are energy fields that oscillate at exceptionally high speeds, surrounded by and interacting with other oscillating energy fields. The idea of "form" becomes very subtle as delineation between objects is an apparition. The universe is one single wave function that can also be said to consist of many wave functions. The universe is composed of a vast and complex set of interacting fields.

But the joy of sensuality and touch can only be experienced when the obvious interconnectedness of physical forms has been forgotten. So, we choose to gloss over the fact that solidity is an illusion afforded to the physical body and its senses.

This forgetting is referred to as *avidyā*[19], and although it is usually translated as "ignorance", it should be not be taken too pejoratively. It is simply a function, an activity, and a decision, made for the specific purpose of enjoying a very focussed existence in space and time. The choice is always there to continue along that path or to choose a more integrative state of being, once the original purpose has been served.

As is well known, the notion of space implies the notion of time. If one wishes to consider one part of space to be separate from another, then the concepts of time, acceleration, and velocity come into play as one must "go" from one virtual fragment to another. Concepts of attainment and loss, yearning and repulsion, also spring into existence.

The idea of tiny particles — of time and matter, that exist upon or within a field, allows the experience and description of linear progression, gradations, and journeys. These "things that change" in space-time is the literal translation of the word *prakṛti*. In this way, it is said that the *puruṣa* experiences *prakṛti*. That which is seen exists for the sake of the seer[20].

---

[19] Yoga Sutras 2.5

[20] Yoga Sutras 2.21

The longer the people stayed playing, the more forgetting occurred. They enjoyed their creations so much in the space they created called "material reality", their behaviour became so repetitive and habitual, that knowledge of their true existence began to fade. The truth became more distant and less frequently recalled, until it slipped out of reach.

When the truth of eternal integration is again apprehended and noticed, one is able to be the whimsical, creative, and blissful over-arching creator of an adventure park called "perceivable material reality projected upon the field of consciousness". On the other hand, when this truth is forgotten, a rather different situation emerges. Feeling trapped, people build strategies to survive in this new situation as a separate and bound individual.

Sometimes, they have an inkling that they have forgotten something very important... Often this semi-tangible intuition is apprehended in dreams, as though just out of reach.

The aim of *sanātan dharma*, and all spiritual practice, is to continue to experience the joy of learning and new experiences and all the great reasons we created this world, while also experiencing the reality of eternal existence beyond our self-created illusions.

You are here because you desire to have it all — to feel the timeless unity and peace of all that is, while also jumping into bespoke experiences. This is *sanātan dharma*. I recall Sharath Jois telling his students in a conference that *yoga* has no starting point and no central teacher. This system is continuous, ever-flowing as humans recall the knowledge.

We can continue to fragment and explore polarities like attraction and aversion, virtue and vice, accumulation and loss, as much as we wish to. We can develop societies and technologies, doctrines and beliefs, allegiance and diversity, sparks of excitement and understanding, all contained within our consciousness. Still, at all times, there is a doorway for anyone who wishes to see what happens when the compulsion to divide consciousness is stopped and reversed.

Indian wisdom centres around this attitude. It is intellectually robust and maintains an incredible diversity and eagerness towards debate, and rebellion against dogma. There is a propensity to not claim personal authorship of wisdom, and a strong awareness of very long lineages[21].

All dialogue is redundant

A tangible way to begin implementing spirituality in everyday life is to consider that mental content can be classified. Indian spiritual practices assist one to notice and classify their mental content. There are many points of view on this, but for now consider two simple classifications.

1. Verbal monologue or dialogue, words and sentences taking the form of descriptions, labels, discussion, either spoken silently in the mind or spoken out loud.

2. Ideas, notions, concepts, visions, inspirations, memories, fantasies, and prompt experiences of understanding that exist non verbally and without description.

When discussion occurs in the mind (type 1 listed above), it does so after an initial instantaneous flash of vision or ideation (type 2). It is quite common for people to be unaware of this visionary aspect of cognition, as it happens so fast and is very quickly followed by long strings of words and verbiage that describe or articulate the vision. People often miss the initial flash and only notice the drawling inner voice that discusses and describes. Many people then believe that the inner talking they hear is the whole mind and that it comes up with ideas, but this is not true.

---

[21] The word Hindu is derived from "Indus", a geographical term referring to the Indus Valley and the civilisations found there. In the 19th century, the British added the suffix "ism" in order to label the "religion" of the people of India, and the word began to lose its geographical association. Really, there is no such thing as "Hinduism". It is a term created in a colonialist context to describe a complex set of beliefs, rituals and customs observed by outsiders.

The poetic notion of revelation is actually how consciousness naturally operates and we can pursue the visionary experience much more than we usually do. The plane where visionary content exists can be viewed, experienced, and sculpted with results that are so pleasant and useful that it forms a self-supporting incentive to stop chattering in your head.

An idea is instantaneous. It comes in a flash, like lightning striking the ground. This is called *pratibhā*. Ideas are easy to miss due to this rapidity, and if you're in the middle of talking to yourself when they appear, they tend to blend into the discussion that you are already having. But you don't have to miss them. You may remain open in the visionary state and see them clearly as they arise.

Buddhist and secular mindfulness meditation (arising from Buddhist techniques) gives people permission to explore quietness, and thus have a greater chance of noticing the plane of visions. Similarly, meta-cognition and psychological theory present a safe way to make inroads that are approved by the mainstream. But there is much more.

If you are only willing to go as far as the currently appointed mystics (in this case, psychologists and neuroscientists) have studied, then you will hit a ceiling fairly quickly. If you are adventurous, curious, and confident in your ability to "not go crazy", you may find yourself going much further.

It is possible to be so entranced with your own inner chatter that you do not recognise the truth of the independence of ideas from dialogue. You may be so enraptured by your inner sentences that you assume the voice is the total you, and that there is nothing else. But if you practice techniques of *yoga*, you will see the truth of ideas and memories and images as occurring in a flash, and the choice that you have to chatter about them in your head, or not.

The words in your head are not your ideas, they are descriptions of your ideas. The inner dialogue is a mechanical function of the brain that "talks about" what is visible in consciousness. There is no new information in your commentary. It is simply a description of content that has become visible in a momentary flash. Ignorance of this fact often leads people to believe that their inner dialogue is the sum total of their mind; their inner dialogue is so noisy that it is identified as the core experience of existence. The images that cause the dialogue are usually forgotten.

The practice of identifying ideas without immediately indulging the habit of chatter is one that *yoga* seeks to explore and develop. We have a reasoning intellect that responds to ideas and creates dialogue in our minds. By all means, analyse your ideas, talk to yourself about them in your head and outside your head. But realise the describing process is different from the receiving of ideas.

It is obviously sometimes necessary to speak about and record ideas with words, so we catch the idea, describe and articulate it. This is a delicate play between two worlds. The idea exists in that nebulous plane, and we then channel it into the plane of words. If you talk too much, you may feel like the original idea slips away. All chattering, be it analysis, reasoning, opining, exists in a different place to that of instantaneous ideas.

Reduce your addiction to talking

Indian thought elaborates on this through the doctrine of speech — known as *vāc*, which means voice, speech, utterance. When teaching people about this technique of classifying mental content, I avoid using English words and new age terms as much as possible. Sanskrit pre-dates English by a long way, and the superimposition of a modern lexicon carries unhelpful baggage. Even the use of Latin and Greek terms creates associations with streams of modern thought that can create misunderstandings.

The habit of nattering to yourself about what appears in your consciousness can be so ingrained and rapid that one can be unaware of any other way to operate. Even after a commitment is made to stop talking and explore subtle consciousness, still it is common to find yourself emerging periodically from a long inner dialogue. But with practice you can live exclusively in the levels above speech.

It is as simple as creating a new habit of catching yourself talking, then stopping, and paying attention to the nebulae of visionary content. Rather than chatting to yourself about your thoughts and feelings, you reside or centre yourself in the place above thought. You are simply aware of forms and movements.

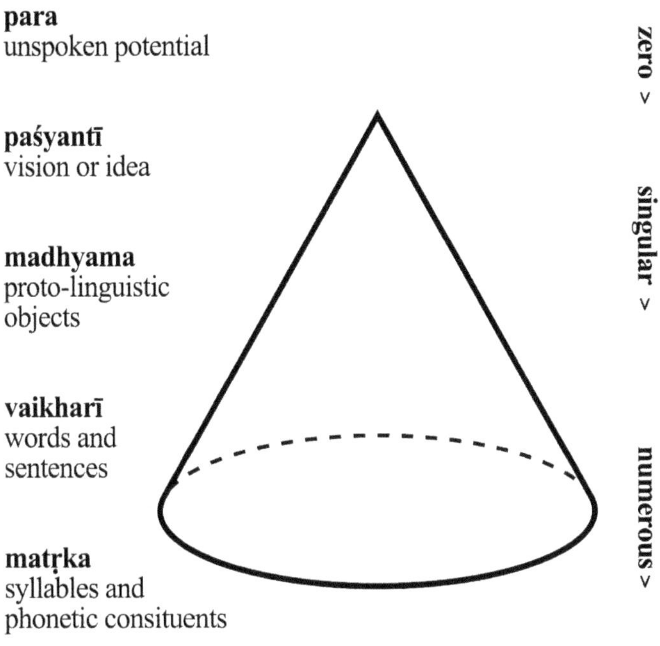

Diagram: the Indian notion of vāc and levels of speech

Practice noticing ideas and then **not** describing them to yourself in your mind. Just relax and hold them there in their native form. Resist the urge to grasp and record them. Trust, and let things come and go. Practice remembering a scene, and watch it for several continuous minutes. Practice silently seeing it in increasing detail. Allow your curiosity to gently move your focus around the scene, without inner verbalisation.

Yoga provides many methods to loosen our grip on conversation and float upwards, where sources and roots are visible. When we cease dropping down in order to record and analyse, we can view nascent ideas for sustained periods and allow them to morph and reveal.

Something even more staggering occurs along this journey — a new simultaneity emerges. We become greater and more expansive in our ability to be in both places at once. We become able to stay at the top of the mountain, witnessing detailed and rich content, while at the same time being able to indulge in wordplay in the physical world. Later we will explore *śāmbhavī mudrā* as a key technique in this regard.

This insight brings about a radical transformation in the mind. Once you have broken the attachment to talking, after a period of stabilisation, you can wilfully attach yourself to the top of the mountain and also venture down the mountain face into specific tasks and sentences, keeping a secure line to the top. The world is full of examples of great scientists and leaders in respectable fields of human endeavour who, having attempted to solve a puzzle or create something using their ordinary analytical mind, eventually received the epiphanic solution when they weren't expecting it.

To be unattached to talking and describing — being instead sensitive to the higher plane — is the preferred operating condition and it is available to us. When this is known and understood, we can go towards that state using the incredible resources that ancient spiritual teachings provide.

Rediscovery

Modern Western culture is rediscovering gems from the ancient sciences. Recall from chapter one the two-stage spiritual process of integration: the repeating cycle of concentrating deeply inwards and then relaxing expansively outwards.

Well, neuroscience is discovering this natural action as well[22], describing it as alternating cycles of:

- the dorsal attention or task-positive network (concentration)
- the default mode network (loose contemplation)

Task-positive activity points the brain down the mountain towards specificity, and this is the bias of humanity at the moment. Default mode activity points the mind upwards to more options and a greater sense of will. Hence the utility of meditative practices to calm a person while awake, yielding imaginative and non-discursive awareness.

As we can see, materialist science catches up with ancient truths over time. It is the trailing edge of evolution, focusing on effects and their immediate causes. A solely empirical approach starts at the level of phenomena and traces up through causes in an iterative fashion. This approach is not enough for us to evolve quickly. For that, we also need visionary ideas and speculation. We need entire populations of inspired people who pursue the highest ideals of science.

---

[22] Silberstein et al., "Dopaminergic modulation of default mode network brain functional connectivity in attention deficit hyperactivity disorder," Brain and Behaviour, Sep 28 2016

Use schools and teachers

Spiritual teachings and organisations can help us if we view them as tools and understand that the real work is one of scientific exploration that we, personally, need to perform. Study under the guidance of the best teacher you can find, one who practices *yoga* in the truest sense that you can identify. Do whatever you can do to be in touch with fertile spiritual endeavour.

Books are useful. Schema and guidelines can be important. But don't do something only because a book or a teacher said to — do it because you are a scientist and an explorer. Make choices that include your sense of interest and curiosity about what happens in your universe. If you find yourself growing and becoming more capable in the world, more sensitive and stable, more loving, then you are on a positive path.

It is easy enough to see how any teaching can become less dynamic, less inspired, and more formalised over time. This is not "bad" as such — and it is certainly not controversial either — it is just what happens when teachings are documented for the purpose of propagation.

The best way to learn something is to be taught in-person. So much non-verbal communication occurs in that context to speed up the process. With interactive face-to-face teaching, teachers can respond and adapt to indications of uncertainty or understanding expressed by students. To record ideas onto paper for a hypothetical future use, by persons unknown, is quite a difficult thing and compromises are frequent.

Revere the reformers

Very often, when a visionary teacher dies and hands over their legacy to their students, the school withers and dies. Sometimes the withering occurs before the death of the teacher as well — all sorts of degradations are possible! Whenever you rely on things written, you must assume there is a limit to the depth of teaching. At times, the rules and dogma must be rattled, and one must "wake up" with a fresh clarity and a new context, armed with amazing resources.

Several times in the recorded history of India, the natural phenomenon of solidification and forgetfulness has been mitigated by reformation.

Back in the 8th century Śrī Śaṅkara, who has been ascribed authorship of Yoga Tārāvalī, arose to expose the ritualism that had accumulated at the hand of the Brahmins of the age[23]. He saw the religiosity and unthinking excess that had arisen in society. In his short life of 30 or so years, he wrote many theses on consciousness and non-dual reality, as well as numerous commentaries on the principal Upanishads. He single-handedly propagated the essential philosophies of India and helped remove dogmatism that had developed in the spiritual institutions, breathing new life into national knowledge. The planet is richer for his contribution.

The great Śrī Aurobindo of the 20th century is a veritable titan, possessing an ethic that saw him produce a swathe of substantive books describing in detail the model of being and evolution stemming from the Upanishads. As a young man he was taken to England to be educated and had a brilliant scholastic career. Upon returning to India, he worked in government for a while before becoming a Nationalist revolutionary of note. He was accused of involvement with bombings, and narrowly escaped conviction on charges of sedition. He ceased political activities after several spiritual experiences and channelled his energy into his teaching of an integral *yoga*[24]. His British education helped him produce material in the English language that are probably the most nuanced and effective works available today. I would be truly thrilled if you were to stop reading this book immediately and instead read his.

---

[23] Scholars note that the text of the Yoga Tārāvalī could be dated to anywhere as late as the 15th century CE. However, there is considerable debate around authorship and attribution in the study of Sanskrit texts, due to authors from particular lineages often sharing or using the same name.

[24] Śrī Aurobindo, *Autobiographical Notes*, 2006

The story of Jiddu Krishnamurti is also very impressive. He was selected as a child to become a spiritual teacher to the world. He possessed extraordinary gifts and was taught and raised with this purpose. When he reached his early 30s, he recognised the folly of building organisational structures and the inevitability of dogmatism when institutionalising spiritual knowledge. He decided to dissolve the organisation that had been preparing for his leadership. He delivered a speech called The Truth is a Pathless Land, in which he explains that truth is limitless and unconditioned, and any attempt to organise it or market it kills it. It becomes a mere creed or religion, objectified for those not strong enough to seek absolute truth[25].

Ashtanga Yoga has a reputation for being tough

Ashtanga Vinyasa Yoga is a system like any other that needs to be periodically shaken and reformed in order to remain dynamic and useful. We often see *yoga* being too rigidly implemented, and this limits access to a beautiful practice of spiritual growth and healing. Rigidity in teaching forces the creation of offshoots or deviations to compensate.

My journey into *yoga* as an adult is an example of what I would consider a masochistic approach, and Ashtanga Yoga has a tendency to attract this kind of person. I very much enjoyed having high standards to work towards. In the early years, I wanted to be on the edge of my capacity (and the edge of injury) at all times. When I studied in the city of Mysore, hanging out with "Ashtangis" from around the world, I recall a significant number of them had conquered, or were conquering, addiction through the practice[26]. It is a fantastic way to channel an energetic persona into something healthy and self-regulating.

---

[25] J. Krishnamurti, "Truth is a Pathless Land," (speech delivered 3 August 1929)

[26] Well known Ashtanga Yoga teachers Jessica and Taylor Hunt have established the Trini Foundation, a non-profit organization dedicated to helping people with addiction to recover using the practice

Having a relatively safe outlet for your enthusiasm is of great value. Ashtanga Yoga in particular comes with a natural unfolding of interoceptive self-awareness, which means that your decisions in life are more keenly felt in your body. The harmful behaviours you indulge are more clearly felt; the healthy behaviours you indulge are more fully enjoyed; and there is a natural balancing as a result.

Simple things like healthy eating tend to occur quite naturally for students of *yoga*, and often without any conscious decision or external prodding. It simply feels better to eat well, so you do. A broad sense of wellbeing begins to outweigh a short-term sugar-high, for example. Students attain a well-rounded and self-generated high.

There are some stunning implementations of Ashtanga Vinyasa Yoga, and they tend to be over-represented in the media because they are so visually impressive. But Mysore style classes are not just for the obsessed, gifted, or professional *yogin*-s. A bespoke and therapeutic approach is not as photogenic as contortion and hand-standing, nevertheless it is the historic backbone of *āsana*. It is true that this practice leads individuals to develop amazing capacities and skills — I never wanted to be able to handstand or put my leg behind my head, but it happened gradually over time.

These feats are prone to catching the eye of popular culture, but I want to reveal that Mysore style is actually a humble and therapeutic form of practice, and that most of the people around the world who practice it do so with a focus on long breaths and competent management of limitations. You can use it as an intense vehicle for transformation, implementing a fervent six days-per-week practice with austerity and fire, or you can use it as a physiotherapy space to explore peace and quiet in the midst of a city.

Perhaps even a dynamic play between the two — the Sanskrit word *līlā* is employed in this context and it means a spontaneous play or drama, even a courtship between the modes of nature. **A Mysore style studio is a research institute full of independent researchers. We use existing ideas as a framework, and as reference material, but not as ideology. Everything is on the table to be employed and questioned.**

Mysore yoga traditions

It is not surprising that such an egalitarian style of *yoga* class sprang so eagerly from the city of Mysore in the state of Karnataka in South India. The ruling Wadiyar royal family consistently demonstrated progressive values. Much is known about the activities of the family during modern history, and local families and scholars eagerly share the virtues and accomplishments of the time.

Mummadi Krishnaraja Wadiyar III ruled from 1799 to 1868. He was a scholar himself and sponsored many other scholars. He composed many works in the Kannada and Sanskrit languages, and was positively influenced by Western concepts of design and architecture. One significant work that he either authored or compiled is named *śrītattvanidhi*, which means The Illustrious Treasure of Realities, and contains illustrations and descriptions of 122 *āsana* of a kind familiar to modern practitioners of *yoga*. It is said that in this age, before the current trend of popular public classes, *yoga* was quiet and private. Those who studied and practiced did so for the purpose of evolution and there was far less emphasis on exercise and general health.

Maharaja Chamarajendra Wadiyar X ruled between 1868 and 1894. He was socially progressive and implemented the first democratic representative assembly in India. He and his family prioritised women's education and equal access to health care regardless of caste. He thought that a rich person ought to expect to be in a hospital bed beside a poor person. They expressed a desire to have the downtrodden brought into the mainstream, something that the upper class opposed.

For generations the Mysore royal family adopted policies and projects that demonstrated an inclusive attitude, and one that provided citizens with opportunities in a rapidly evolving world. During this period, the state became the first in Asia to generate hydroelectric power. They provided English and Sanskrit language education, created housing and temples, provided indoor games for the population, and prioritised wildlife preservation. They were strong advocates of the arts (Wadiyar X was a violinist himself) and they made education along these lines available to far more people than the national culture usually permitted.

Wadiyar X died of sudden illness in 1894 at the age of 31, and for the next eight years his wife Kempa Nanjammani Vani Vilasa Sannidhana ruled the kingdom as *maharani*, until their son came of age and became maharaja. Despite her personal grief from losing her husband at such a young age, she stepped into the position with courage and persistence. She ruled amongst the great sadness across the entire country at the loss of Wadiyar X, a time of grief exacerbated by a plague that wiped out half of the population of the district.

Great progress was made in the area with the electricity and water supply growing along with other building works. It is said that during this period, the city of Mysore became the first in India to have electric street lighting. The queen-regent conducted herself with such grace and discipline in this difficult period that she became known as one of the jewels in the history of Mysore.

In 1902 her son took over the kingdom. Krishna Raja Wadiyar IV continued the family tradition of honouring the populace. He considered himself as property of the populace, rather than a ruler. During his reign he continued the family work to reduce poverty and to increase access to education. Visitors from Britain and America heaped praise on the king over his years. Many colleges were opened in this time, including the Science College for Women and the University of Mysore, agricultural schools, along with factories, dams, mills, and hospitals.

During the reign of Krishna Raja Wadiyar IV, a fellow named Tirumalai Krishnamacharya began to teach *yoga* in Mysore. Krishnamacharya had studied *yoga* seven and a half years, in a cave at the foot of Mount Kailash, with Ramamohana Brahmachari. The teacher-student dynamic was already a little untraditional, as Krishnamacharya had requested that he be allowed to spend three months per year with the viceroy of Simla, who he had treated for diabetes and who had assisted him with his travels[27].

[27] A. G. Mohan, *Krishnamacharya: His Life and Teachings* (Boulder: Shambhala Publications, 2010)

Tradition was even more significantly altered Krishnamacharya's studies were finished. At this time, Brahmachari instructed Krishnamacharya to participate in householder life — to live as a married man in a city and teach *yoga* in that context, to regular people. The numbers of aspirants seeking to live in the mountains and be taught in this way had been falling, and there was a risk that the knowledge would be lost, so the trend was emerging for *guru*-s to adopt lifestyles more connected with the householder experience.

Krishnamacharya had such a prodigious yearning for knowledge that even after his time in the mountains he continued to pursue tertiary education in many fields of Indian thought. He studied the sacred texts and received degrees at several philosophical schools. All the while, he was practicing *āsana* and *prāṇāyāma* that his father had taught him as a child. As a young man, he travelled in search of higher education and master teachers. Along the way, he gathered support and scholarships by proving himself to those in positions of authority, and by attracting lucky situations.

He was 37 years old when he decided that his studies were finally complete and that it was time to seriously address the instructions of his *guru*. His decision to teach *yoga* troubled his family, as it would be easy for him to have a more respectable role in an institution. He knew that things would work out if he followed the directions of his teacher. Soon enough, the king of Mysore invited him to teach at Mysore Palace.

Krishnamacharya pioneered what we have come to know as *yoga* in the form of syllabi and classes. He created and taught tailored sequences and techniques that improved the health of people. He taught the adults and royal family in private consultations about basic *āsana* and *prāṇāyāma*, while the youth were taught sequences of postures that look familiar to us, and that were later published.

He had the same attitude as the royal family in terms of religion, in that he held his own understandings but also supported others with their own. He adapted his teaching for Hindus, Muslims, Christians, and atheists. This allowed him to be sought out as a proficient spiritual teacher and authority, and to this end he continued to travel and lecture while running the *yoga* school in Mysore. He made a name for himself by demonstrating the stopping of his heart, and by teaching women. The first Westerner he ever taught was a woman named Indra Devi.

Krishnamacharya's work eventually solidified into set sequences and structures that were then modified and proliferated by a few key students.

One such student, BKS Iyengar, developed an alternative approach. Rather than emphasising the flowing linkage of many movements with breath, he instead focused on strict alignment and muscular activations in each pose.

Another student, Pattabhi Jois, retained the method of *vinyāsa* taught by Krishnamacharya, where postures are connected together with precise transitions. It is known as Ashtanga Vinyasa Yoga, or Ashtanga Yoga. Pattabhi Jois continued to develop the sequences over a few decades of experimentation. His children (Manju and Saraswathi) and grandchildren (Sharath and Sharmilla), continue to teach their interpretations of Ashtanga Vinyasa Yoga around the world.

Yet another student, BNS Iyengar (note a different Iyengar to BKS), teaches a style similar to what we know as the Ashtanga Vinyasa style of the Jois family that contains greater emphasis on *prāṇāyāma*.

Śrīvatsa Ramaswami is one of the last students of Krishnamacharya. He comprehensively documented the teachings and named the style Vinyasa Krama. He presents *āsana* grouped into anatomical themes and describes their practice with an emphatic adherence to *vinyāsa*, that is, entering and exiting poses with a particular combination of breath and movement[28].

All styles of *yoga* come with sets of rules. Typically, such rules exist for reasons of anatomical and psychological safety. In more recent decades we see the emergence of another kind of rule — a convention that exists to help teachers manage large classes. As Westerners flocked to India, there was a need to experiment with ways to manage potentially hundreds of students practicing in the one *yoga* school each day.

---

[28] S. Ramaswami, *The Complete Book of Vinyasa Yoga* (Boston: Da Capo Press 2005)

A pertinent example of procedural rule relates to when a student is permitted to attempt a new pose and incorporate it into their routine. In a traditionally intimate class environment, there would be individual assessment of students and bespoke instruction on when to begin practicing new poses, and what those poses ought to be, and alignment cues to suit the individual body type. In a large modern class with hundreds of people visiting from all around the world, such rules help teachers manage the volume of students. If a teacher wants to service so many students at once, there simply will not be time to analyse and speak to each one thoroughly, so guidelines arise.

Sometimes, these guidelines become adopted as permanent edicts, and this is unhelpful and demonstrates the freezing effect of systemisation. We must not let this occur. As discussed, systemisation involves solidification into ordered forms. Elements can become more rigid and less dynamic. Secondary interpretations arise and separation from the original vision occurs. There is no single source of truth — look at the number of lineage holders who exist, listed above, let alone the many Western teachers who have studied under the greats of India.

Mutiny

Master of *yoga* and Kashmir Shaivism, I.K. Taimni, speaks of accretions of tradition[29] that form around the kernel of actual truths. With the passage of time, he says, proponents arrive who have often lost touch with the realities of truths that they expound, and there becomes a greater interest in **enforcement** than of direct realisation of spiritual knowledge.

It is inevitable that rules are broken. Sometimes they are broken due to immaturity and impatience, but sometimes it follows a rational assessment of the situation and a difference of context or opinion. In any case, I would go as far as to say that most popular forms of flowing *yoga* in the West today have been invented by disgruntled former students of Ashtanga Vinyasa Yoga! The more recently created styles of *yoga* have often been forced into

[29] I.K. Taimni, *Science and Occultism* (Adyar: Vasanta Press 1974)

existence by dogmatism that prevents people from experimenting. Those who will not tolerate being held back by immovable rules will naturally break away and invent styles that suit their own experience and the real-world experience of their students.

The irony is that in breaking away from dogma and setting up a new set of rules, it is possible for teachers repeat the cycle by seeking to brand their new version of *yoga*, to restrict and control it.

All of this reinforces the need for a *yoga* class format where people are encouraged to explore with a sense of personal authority and freedom, informed by expert advice and all manner of supporting knowledge, and this is what happens in a progressive Mysore style environment.

Thrive, go beyond better

Of course, rigid enforcement of statutory rules happens across all sectors of human society. Social conditioning values conformity to rules. Entry to society presupposes the personal adoption of external systems of values, and the ceding of some agency to the organisations and institutions which govern us as a group. In modern psychology, this concept is called the external locus of control — and this can cause a sense of powerlessness that is associated with negative behaviours and poor mental health.

There is a bleak and materialist point of view in the modern world, which informs people that they are nothing but flesh robots with an emergent quirk known as the mind. These minds are poor and untrustworthy pieces of equipment, which struggle to control the savage human genetic hardware of the brain/body complex — given half a chance we would apparently revert to a throwback state of violence and rape and murder.

This view, which emphasises recent evidence about the nature of biology and evolution over other understandings of the human being, is used as a comfortable lens to view the past, allowing us to believe that we have reached our peak. Anything that contradicts this charmingly linear story of development is ignored. This includes evidence of advanced civilisations during ancient times, research into unified consciousness that dissolves seemingly solid boundaries between individuals, and more. Uncomfortable truths of mind affecting matter are documented, given labels like "placebo", and pushed aside.

This worldview doubles down on the alleged insignificance of mind, finding proof that it is inherently untrustworthy and cannot be relied upon for evidence. Children are informed that "they only use 20% of their brains" and must rely on voices other than their own for a sense of truth, happiness, and even for survival. Society staggers onwards towards consumerism and nihilism.

I will draw your attention to the fact that we can go much further in the positive direction. Recall *sanātan dharma,* remember your true nature. You were born wise. You were born clairvoyant. We can do better than this. Why do we not insist upon the complete and utter flourishing of individuals and species, the ecstatic evolution of humanity and the planet? It is common to foster counter-productive assumptions. Beliefs around scarcity, the virtue of suffering, lack of personal influence are popular, still they remain beliefs.

We could insist that every person be raised and live in an environment where it is natural and easy to bounce out of a clean bed each morning and embrace a joyous existence of creative play. Each person developing their own intuition, sense of personal authorship, bolstered by a planet full of parental figures.

Creativity, spontaneity, and joy are three parts of one thing. So, if you are seeking joy, seek spontaneity. Good ideas happen in a flash! Impulses for fun and play appear when conditions are loose, when there is free time, when there is mobility and dynamism in body and mind.

There can be no spontaneity when the bulk of each day is scripted and the time for play is an allocated block that is accessible only after other more mechanical duties are completed.

The hero's journey is to stretch

We must surge upward, individually and collectively. It is difficult to use our imagination when artificial constructs wall us in. The child-like ease falls away and we forget that we ever had an imagination that can be used to create reality.

If it seems hard to use your imagination to clearly visualise the desired future, your highest ideals for yourself and the community — good! Keep going. It will stretch your brain and your creative capacity. When surrounded by walls, one at least has many reminders to go beyond.

It could even be considered easier with such constrictions littered through society. Everywhere there is a limit being imposed, thus everywhere there is a reminder that you are the true author of this story and that everything you see is raw material for you to use.

The commercial drive toward mere symptom-relief infiltrates new age therapies as well as allopathic medicine. Instead of a defensive focus on healing and coping, instead of analysing the reasons why you feel you cannot express yourself, get on with the job of flourishing. Instead of sifting through your flaws, construct something new. You don't have to analyse and debug everything that's "wrong" with you.

The amazing quality of life is that you grow by reaching up to the sky, not by looking at where you came from. You are a refinery, a transformer of raw material. Everything within is to be converted to a higher form. Accept the sunlight and water and soil, cast your gaze up to the sky, and trust that everything you need is at hand and always will be.

Standing on the shoulders of giants

There are always numerous reasons to stay at home and avoid what you really want to do, to choose a sideways movement instead of a bold step forward. You will be supported by vast numbers of people and corporate entities who will join you in maligning the efforts of those who do wish to soar beyond the ordinary. We know that disempowered consumers are far more valuable, far more likely to repeatedly consume.

I remember working in a corporate office, being pudgy and deciding to lose weight. I started visibly exercising in my lunch breaks, and a rather unfit colleague said these words to me, without an iota of irony or humour: "don't you know that exercise is a leading cause of injury?"

It's staggering even today the logic in this statement: if you use your body, it might go wrong, so don't. This fellow did not pursue exercise and found evidence in popular media to support his apathy. In the same office on a different day, I was observed eating an enormous bowl of vegetables and another colleague said to me: "You shouldn't eat that; cauliflower gives you gout". There will always be a valid-seeming reason to stay sedentary, to resist the evolution that you deeply want.

See the positive contribution of eons of humans who have toiled, invested, and sacrificed themselves in pursuits that have allowed us to arrive right here and right now. Look at what they did, look at the high vantage we find ourselves privileged to possess. We have been gifted such an accumulation of riches and knowledge.

Our potential in life is immense. Consider the well-known Latin phrase *nanos gigantum humeris insidentes*, which translates to "standing on the shoulders of giants", a metaphor for discovering truth by building on previous discoveries.

Yoga is sometimes framed as something that will help you cope, but I recommend allowing the idea of coping to fall away as you invigorate your imagination and trust that everything you need will come in due time and that anything you experience along the way is a purely positive step along the path.

The first section of the Ashtanga Vinyasa Yoga opening chant, which is recited by groups of *yoga* students each morning, is taken from the first śloka of the Sanskrit text called Yoga Tārāvalī. This title translates as "cosmic waves of integration" or "an array of stars about *yoga*".

The first verse, or *śloka*, of the text shown below is an acknowledgement of the contribution of all the enthusiasts that have preceded us, and for us to aspire to grow into our ideals. This chant itself is a great example of a synthetic approach to *yoga* — one half is taken from Yoga Tārāvalī, attributed to Śrī Śaṅkara, while the other is from the Kūrma Purāṇa.

Here is the first verse:

वन्दे गुरूणां चरणारविन्दे संदर्शितस्वात्मसुखावबोधे |
जनस्य ये जाङ्गलिकायमाने संसार हालाहल मोहशान्त्यै ||

vande gurūṇāṃ caraṇāravinde saṁdarśitasvātmasukhāvabodhe
janasya ye jāṅgalikāyamāne saṃsāra hālāhala mohaśāntyai

I revere this, the vision of the true Self, which is revealed at the feet of the guru-s. It causes the joyful condition and all the good things. It is the snake-charmer that neutralises deadly poison of false-identity, the delusion of samsara, for the peace of humanity.

The line "I bow to the lotus feet of my revered preceptor" is not disempowering and it is not religious. Your ultimate guide, that which "removes darkness", is your own highest Self — your searchlight.

This is the part of you that spans a greater quantity of time and space. It can see further afield than the mundane mind. It is that which you have access to in increasing measure, with practice.

When we chant, we are reminding ourselves to commit to our ideals, and then employ the physical practice of stretching and expanding as a vehicle of positive reinforcement that builds upon itself exponentially.

By chanting this invocation, we remind ourselves to invest time and effort and concentration to stretch ourselves to that place. We ask the basic physical brain to lay down its defences and suspend its fear of anything that seems alien.

Taken in a sceptical context, surrender and devotion like this can connote weakness and incredulity. In the context of *yoga*, this is a quality encompassing fearlessness, trust, and confidence.

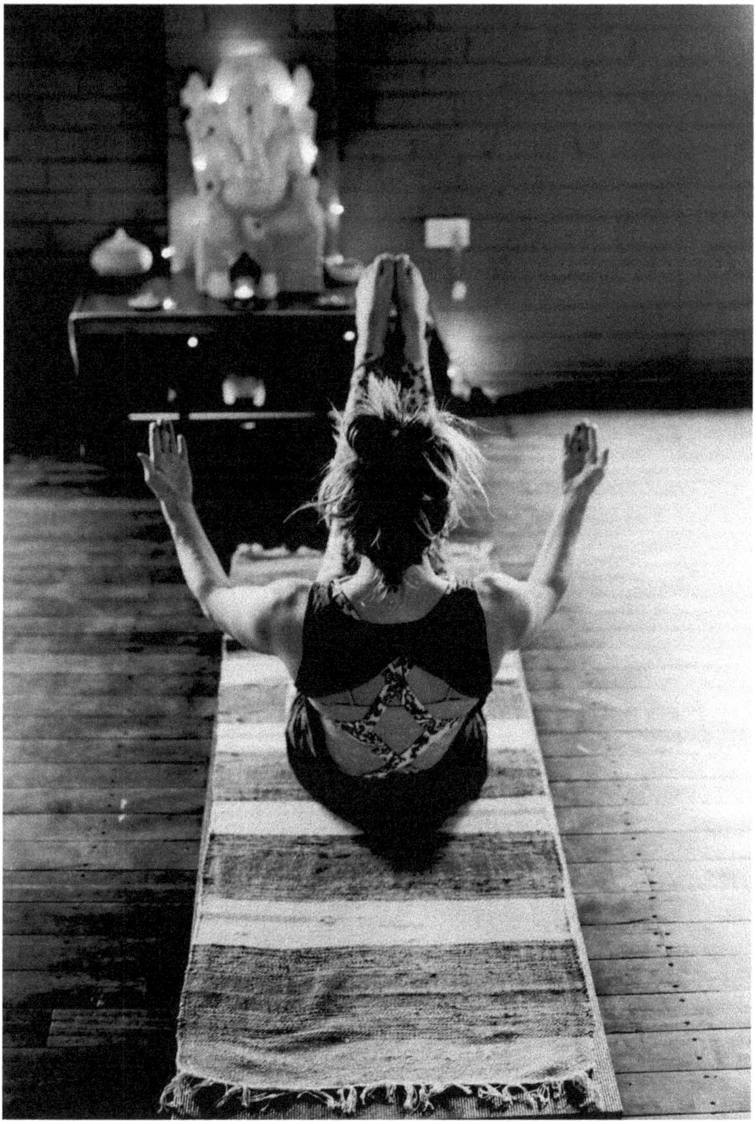

Photo credit: Ash Wheelhouse

4

YOGA THERAPY

The question is often asked: how can I remember and retain states of exalted inspiration where I seem to have a better perspective and feel more energised? Why do I seem to go through cycles of losing this perspective and slipping back into a mundane or reactive behaviour, only to eventually come around and remember again that state of expanded realisation I was so adamant I would keep?

The way to avoid this cycle of forgetting and remembering is to include the physical body in your psychological and spiritual journey.

There is often segregation within an individual. The spiritual, mental, and physical worlds (use any method of subdivision you like) are fenced off from one another and experienced in a piecemeal fashion. It is possible for the physical body to even be disparaged or devalued, in favour of mental and spiritual aspects. Sometimes people will pursue a meditation practice to the detriment of the body, or vice versa. Mysore style classes balance this tendency and lead to integration — *yoga* itself.

The body can act as an anchor or a kite

If you wish your mind to be clear and joyous, if you wish to retain high mental states, then the body must come along for the ride. Your body can be your best friend, tapping you on the shoulder, releasing helpful neurotransmitters, delivering intuitive guidance, facilitating effortless play in life. Or it can be a nuisance, a complaining pest.

Your posture affects your attitude — this is well known. Positive body posture has been shown to have a corresponding effect on mood, memories and associations[30]. When you walk down the street with a positive body posture, you are more likely to notice positive aspects of the world around you.

It is crucial for a human to know innately that they are fit and healthy. Consider the assurance that one might feel if they instinctively know they are athletic enough to sprint after a wayward child and save them from sudden danger. Consider the confidence of a person who takes it for granted that if they trip over, the landing will be nothing more than a funny anecdote — the condition of being playfully buffeted by nature.

Freedom in the physical body is more important than material wealth. To be fragile in the bones and joints is to live inside a shaky home. For some people, tripping over in the garden would have dire consequences. For some, it can even hurt to breathe deeply.

Limitation in the body accumulates very slowly most of the time, and it often tracks along with chronological age, so it is often assumed that tightness is a **result** of age. But it is not. Tightness is a result of behaviour and **lack of** activity. There are many people who are willing and able to make healthy physicality a core part of their entire lives who experience a continual **increase** of bodily capacity and enjoyment as they age.

---

[30] E. Peper et al., "How Posture Affects Memory Recall and Mood," Biofeedback, April 2017

It may not be **common** — society does not always help us prioritise in this way — but it is easy enough to find proof of concept.

Is it any wonder people feel like they are dying as they age? Their freedom is slowly being withdrawn. It does not have to be this way. When you can stand up tall and throw your shoulders back and laugh loudly without hesitation or pain, then you can thrive. You are unrestricted. If you can lift a child and throw them in the air and catch them easily, then you demonstrate a fun and joyous attitude that is self-sustaining. Surely this is the baseline we need to enjoy life.

Begin by creating bodily freedom through *āsana*, and note that it is done by the individual student, not by anyone else. The teacher is a helper on the side, not a doctor or a saviour. Far from any religiosity, *yoga* is centred in self-responsibility, autonomy, and authorship.

Such authority comes with the integration of those segregated pieces of one's totality. With *āsana* and the practice of structured breathing called *prāṇāyāma*, we can experience more aspects of ourselves simultaneously. Doing so makes us smarter and happier. Rather than working to ignore pain and discord, rather than denying access to our latent talents, all can be brought into the sunshine of our conscious awareness — and it feels good.

Recall again the Western biological concept of interoception — the perception of inner bodily sensations. This is a modern term that encapsulates many aspects of Mysore style Ashtanga Yoga. It is a quiet and fluid physical practice of opening and closing the ribcage, flexing and extending the spine and all other joints, and breathing deeply and rhythmically. It enhances interoception as the senses are expanded into all the corners of the body. This phenomenon was established by the *yogin*-s of lore who were able to modify automatic functions of the body.

Modern research indicates that interoception has a crucial role in "body ownership" and "selfhood[31] [32] , which is a formal way of saying that all of one's experience is invited into a large and whole sense of self. This has direct bearing on the sense of agency, of personal ability and responsibility, as well as multisensory integration — the complete and real-time processing of sensory data. Interoceptive ability is also linked to intuitive judgment and decision-making[33] [34], emotional experience[35] [36] , emotional processing[37] [38] , behavioural self-regulation[39] and body image[40] [41]. Put simply, higher interoceptive ability means faster recognition of mental, physical and internal stimuli and therefore increases the ability of a person to manage them promptly.

---

[31] A. Seth, "Interoceptive inference, emotion, and the embodied self," Trends in Cognitive Sciences, Vol. 17, Issue 11, Nov 01 2013

[32] M. Tsakiris, A. Tajadura-Jiménez, M. Costantini, "Just a heartbeat away from one's body: Interoceptive sensitivity predicts malleability of body-representations," Proceedings of the Royal Society B, Aug 22 2011

[33] B. Dunn et al., "Listening to Your Heart: How Interoception Shapes Emotion Experience and Intuitive Decision Making," Psychological Science

[34] N Werner et al., "Enhanced cardiac perception is associated with benefits in decision-making," Psychophysiology, 12 Oct 2009

[35] O. Pollatos et al., "Heart rate response after emotional picture presentation is modulated by interoceptive awareness," International Journal of Psychophysiology, Vol. 63, January 2007

[36] S. Wiens, E. Mezzacappa, E. Katkin, "Heartbeat detection and the experience of emotions," Cognition and Emotion, Vol. 14, 2000

[37] L. Maister, T. Tang, M. Tsakiris, "Neurobehavioral evidence of interoceptive sensitivity in early infancy," Elife, 8 Aug 2017

[38] Y. Terasawa, M, Shibata, Y. Moriguchi, S. Umeda, "Anterior insular cortex mediates bodily sensibility and social anxiety," Social Cognitive and Affective Neuroscience. 13 Sep 2012

[39] B. Herbert, P. Ulbrich, R. Schandry, "Interoceptive sensitivity and physical effort: Implications for the self-control of physical load in everyday life", Psychophysiology 07 Feb 2007

[40] D. Badoud, M. Tsakiris, "From the body's viscera to the body's image: Is there a link between interoception and body image concerns?" Neuroscience & Biobehavioral Reviews, Vol. 77, June 2017

[41] G. Zamariola et al., "Can you feel the body that you see? On the relationship between interoceptive accuracy and body image," Body Image, Vol. 20 Mar 2017

When you can "feel a feeling coming" at a very early stage, as you might see a form appear on the horizon, you can manage it. You can implement reappraisal strategies and sculpt your moment-to-moment experience. On the other hand, when you find yourself overwhelmed by feelings, with a longer delay between their initial presence and your eventual conscious awareness of them, they seem to have suddenly come out of nowhere and it's not as easy to wind them back.

Yoga equips us to be more proactive in shaping our conscious state by increasing this interoceptive sense. Our freedom of will and personal capacity to make good decisions is increased. When emotions are noticed early, as partially-formed inklings, tones, or primordial energy ready to be shaped, they can be allowed to sprout in any manner desired.

A lot of work has been done studying maladies associated with disturbed interoceptive functioning, but only a little has been revealed by modern science about how to develop it and improve access to it.

Some studies indicate that physical posture itself affects interoception, with strong and powerful poses enhancing it[42]. Other studies of groups who display above average abilities are intriguing. Ballet dancers are one such group; the authors of one study emphasise that the process of eliciting emotional states and then attending to and expressing them physically is a factor that enhances interoceptive abilities[43]. Similarly, trained musicians[44] have been shown to have greater interoceptive accuracy than non-musicians, and the integration of auditory, visual and kinaesthetic sense has been identified as a probable reason for this.

---

[42] F. Weineck et al., "Improving interoceptive ability through the practice of power posing: A pilot study," PLOS ONE, 7 Feb 2019

[43] Christensen JF, Gaigg SB, Calvo-Merino B. "I can feel my heartbeat: dancers have increased interoceptive accuracy," Psychophysiology, 21 Sep 2018

[44] Schirmer-Mokwa KL, Fard PR, Zamorano AM, Finkel S, Birbaumer N, Kleber BA, "Evidence for enhanced interoceptive accuracy in professional musicians," Frontiers in Behavioral Neuroscience, 17 Dec 2015

Use a thorn to remove a thorn

There is a strong tendency in some spiritual circles to deny the existence of the world and the body, claiming it to be an illusion. But the world is real, and so is your imagination, and so is the Self. They may not be *what you had previously thought they were*, but they are real. There is indeed an illusory quality to our perceptions, an incompleteness. But the more we learn, the more we see what was previously unseen, and the greater the capacity we have in which to view all things.

A friend of mine who likes to argue against spirituality cites the example of a fellow he once lived with who would sit in a closet under the stairs and meditate for most of his waking hours each day. I have to agree with him in this case — what kind of a life is that?

The physical practices of *yoga* establish clear vision of the body so that it may be used well and enjoyed. There is an old saying that the best way to remove a thorn is to use a thorn. Here we use the body and its problematic trigger of physical tightness and limitation — the thorn — to remove the false notion of limitation altogether.

Studies of interoception support the view that bodily practices, not just meditation practices, are crucial for enhancing interoception. Interestingly, it has been shown that experienced meditators do not show the same above average inner sensitivity as dancers and musicians, contrary to expectations. The meditators' confidence was higher, but their ability to sense the heartbeat was no better than non-meditators[45].

Another study showed that meditators demonstrated enhanced emotional clarity and greater calm, yet were still not able to detect the heartbeat better than non-meditators[46]. This is a consistent finding, that meditators display lower levels of anxiety, but no improvement in interoception[47].

---

[45] Khalsa SS, Rudrauf D, Damasio AR, Davidson RJ, Lutz A, Tranel D. "Interoceptive awareness in experienced meditators," Psychophysiology, 20 May 2008

[46] Nielsen L, Kaszniak AW, "Awareness of subtle emotional feelings: a comparison of long-term meditators and nonmeditators," Emotion. 2006

[47] Melloni M, Sedeño L, Couto B, Reynoso M, Gelormini C, Favaloro R, et al. "Preliminary evidence about the effects of meditation on interoceptive sensitivity and social cognition," Behavioral and Brain Functions. 23 Dec 2013

Physical activity is required to enhance interoception. Ideally one that is self-paced, quiet, centred around deep breathing, with a consistent set of postures and a lack of external distraction (such as music or a teacher's constant instructions). This invariably leads one into a deeper state of self-awareness, and this is where Mysore style *yoga* shines.

Sitting under the stairs, feeling calm, is not the purpose of life. This echoes the warnings given by ancients who maintain that the practice of deep meditation ought not be pursued in isolation — the student must also be established in *āsana*, *prāṇāyāma*, and the behavioural controls called *yama* and *niyama*. The mind must be trained to automatically reside in the state of "active harmony", called *sattva*.

Without this training, there will be a tendency during meditation to fall into either apathy or obsession. In the former case, the effect would be to fall asleep or allow the physical life to become drab and passive, full of empathy but lacking vigour. In the latter case, the effect is to increase the concentration of aggression and lust.

You are here right now, living in time and space and physical existence. The purpose of *yoga* is to simultaneously remain here and yet also access places that are not so obvious — places in your body that are tight or knotted, as well as places in your consciousness that have been forgotten or obscured.

The idea is to positively expand yourself to cover more space and more domains, to heal anything that is in need, rather than to escape. With *yoga*, you are empowered as a scientist and a seer, and with Mysore style classes you can experiment using the many tools on offer.

A tale of three series

The practice of Ashtanga Vinyasa Yoga puts the practitioner on a trajectory towards the unfolding of vision and heightened control over the nervous system. The first step on this path is the application of therapy to the physical body.

When *āsana* is practiced in a Mysore style setting, as opposed to a led class, the student receives many benefits: tailored sequences of movements from experts, physical adjustments from same, and the ability to be self-paced and manage fatigue. The chief attainment of each posture is stability and smooth breathing, and they are arranged in an intelligently designed series that contain movements and counter-movements, intended to facilitate a gradual and safe, whole-body evolution.

This is a hugely positive process; the true inner resource being accessed is the student's own dedication to the task. Secondary to this is advice from the teacher, and implicit or explicit support from other students.

There are three classic series of postures in Ashtanga Vinyasa Yoga, with the final set being vast and most difficult to attain.

1. The primary series is for *yoga* therapy, called *yoga cikitsā*
2. The intermediate series is for energy purification, *nadī śodhana*
3. The advanced series is for demonstration, *sthira bhāga*

A strong foundation is key. The primary series gives the body and mind a routine of poses and techniques to cultivate the right propensities.

But first, Sūrya Namaskāra

Even before a purpose-built series of postures is performed comes the opening movements, called *sūrya namaskāra*, or sun salutations.

If you were to do only one physical *yoga* practice in your life, it would surely be the sun salutations, and there are many people for whom this is their sole practice. Esteemed teacher David Garrigues speaks of spending the first ten years of his journey practicing sun salutations only. The case could absolutely be made that if one did only this over the course of one's life, without any other *āsana*, it would comprise a complete application of the principles of *haṭha yoga* (the word *haṭha* means to use physical effort).

Sun salutations can be an extremely clarifying and energising practice. This short set of fundamental movements contains just about everything needed to maintain a healthy forward bend and back bend, hip mobility, core and upper body strength, and an increasingly large lung capacity[48].

During *sūrya namaskāra* we overwhelm the downward facing tendency of the material mindset. Upward facing dog, *ūrdhva mukha śvānāsana*, is a reversal of sighing expiration. Stretching the inhale intentionally stretches our life. Stretching the chest is an act of trailblazing rebellion to the subliminal urgings of the world of advertising and fear-based news media to cower, hunch, and slink away from our positive and playful nature.

The breath is the pivot point between the conscious and unconscious; it can be both consciously controlled and unconsciously controlled. It is one of the rare functions that straddles the total being in this way.

In *yoga* we put positive energy into our breath, we psychically connect to our breath and silently affirm our existence beyond the mundane.

---

[48] Sharath Jois explained that extremes of mind affect the breath and likewise moderating the breath smooths the mental modes. He said that *sūrya namaskāra* builds great lung capacity, although it takes time, and that a beginner might require 50 breaths to do a sun salutation instead of the ideal 9 breaths.

We connect with the trees, the animals, the human ancestors, the future humans. "I inhale as a unified being" or "I breathe as the eternal and infinite intelligence which is made visible." This can be silently uttered with **every single breath.**

Sūrya *namaskāra* is occurring all the time in daily life, if only slightly. With every inward breath, the chest lifts, the ribs flare out, and the sacrum counter-nutates. With every outward breath the chest drops, the shoulders move forward, and the sacrum moves into nutation. We want to train this natural movement for some time each day, so that for the rest of the day the function is enhanced.

So valuable is this simple set of movements that when one moves onto the primary series, a half sun salutation — called a "jump back" — is performed. This short package of movements is interspersed throughout the series to keep warmth in the body and to reset the spine and mind.

It is repetitive, rhythmic, and incorporates a boisterous pumping action in the lungs along with a full body flexion and extension. It delivers an uplifting charge of energy in between each pose and is sometimes referred to as a *vinyāsa*. When poses are linked like this, there is an incredible blending of the objectives of *āsana*.

The primary series is Yoga Therapy

Should you wish to do more than sun salutations, the various series of Ashtanga Vinyasa Yoga can be employed as a framework and as a general starting point. The primary series is also described with the term *cikitsā*, which means therapy. This sequence of postures contains an effective and fairly complete set of bodily movements that can serve a person very well in undoing the harmful effects of chair sitting and sedentary lifestyles. This blueprint is a sensible, effective, and adjustable series of bone rotations that reworks every joint in the human body. Most of the poses are held in a static fashion for five or more smooth and even breaths.

In Mysore style practice, the standing poses and seated poses of the primary series usually form the starting point. This is also the go-to series for sorting out the body in times of need. When travelling and spending a lot of time sitting, even advanced students will revert to this sequence. It features lots of therapeutic forward bends, twists, and a healthy toning of the core and upper body. The basic therapy of this sequence also helps a great deal for people engaged in careers that involve manual labour and lifting.

With the primary series, the pelvic floor is developed a great deal, and healthy baseline movement patterns are established. Everything starts here and we maintain this series to some extent through the course of our life. This series has a defined purpose and utility and will serve the student well in many ways.

It is possible to perform it in ways that are unsustainable, of course. Excessive strictness or bloody-mindedness can work against our progress. A flexible mindset that permits modifications is essential[49].

Practices change over time like a concertina

As you continue to practice, strength and flexibility increase. At times, a plateau is felt where things feel substantially easier, where you don't really have to stretch much anymore to do a certain pose. Where there was previously a lot of effort, a lot of warming up, now you can do it surprisingly well. It's as though the shape of your joints has changed.

This is the point where the teacher will start adding poses to challenge the student. If the student is still learning the primary series, then more poses from primary will be added. If the student is ready to move beyond the primary series, then poses from intermediate will be added to the end of the primary series, right before the closing sequence.

---

[49] On the topic of strictness, Sharath Jois has said that it takes time, that one should not rush to perfect the practice. He recommended taking extra breaths when a pose is found to be particularly difficult. He said that focusing too much on one *āsana* will result in a loss of heat and therefore flexibility (Conference notes, Mysore 2014)

The total duration of practice will grow and there will eventually be a need to remove easier postures from the tail end so that there is a more reasonable total practice duration. In this way, the sequence expands and contracts like a concertina.

Sometimes teachers assert certain rules dictating minimum durations and prerequisite attainments before moving on to second series or certain other poses. These rules ought to be treated as guidelines. Most of the time they can be traced back to the practical necessities of systemising the practice in a busy school, and it would be irrational to insist upon their strict adherence for their own sake.

In a typical cycle, a student will be working on a sequence of poses that are challenging and that require a concerted effort to reach. The teacher eventually observes that a student has become self-reliant and stable in the breath. The outward physical expression of exertion reduces and is replaced by ease. The student is ready to have more challenging postures added to their practice. This is the oft-quoted *sthirā* and *sukha* that the Yoga Sūtras of Patañjali recommends[50].

The cumulative effect of practicing these sequences is that the joints of the body develop both strength and flexibility in equal measure on all angles. Biases are worked out, and capacity is enhanced without creating new imbalances. Much of the remodelling occurs within the fascia of the body.

Fascia is the organ of interoception

The skin is our largest organ, and it is an organ of **perception**, while fascia is our under-the-surface organ of **interoception**. It is an incredibly strong network of tissue that provides a stable structure within which we have bones, muscles, and organs.

---

[50] Yoga Sutras 2.46

When you see the shape of a person, you are seeing the form of their fascia. Like the wrapping of bandage around an Egyptian mummy, it is a weaved bodysuit, and each tug on one part of the suit affects the whole suit. Fascia contains a dense network of nerve endings as well. Strength, balance, and flexibility are all intertwined in the health of this organ.

Ideally our fascia is pliable and can flex and slide over itself. However, with insufficient movement, the smooth and lubricated nature of a young person's fascia can eventually become littered with stickiness. Tight spots, knots, and adhesions arise, causing disfunction in certain movements. This accumulates to form whole-of-body imbalances, and symptoms can arise in seemingly unrelated parts of the body. Any effort to treat pain and imbalances ought to include a whole-body practice of dynamic stretching and strengthening combined with deep breathing. Treatment of isolated body parts can only go so far.

Just as we overcome psychological conditions from the past — childhood struggles, trauma, bleak world-views — and replace them with habits of aspiration, positive imagination, so too can we evolve our bodies to handle tasks that align with our higher will.

Sometimes when we practice *yoga* poses, we seem to experience the ability to stretch a part of the body easily. We move into a pose and breathe deeply and wait a little while, and we seem to be able to move more freely after a few moments. This is the easy work, stretching muscles, basic mobilisation.

Other times, we appear to reach a hard limit where we just cannot stretch any further. This is the limit imposed by bones and connective tissue. The term "compression" has become very popular in Western *yoga* as a way of explaining that certain people cannot and will not be able to do certain movements. At some point the shape of bones will in fact limit the movement of the body, but there is an extraordinary degree of remodelling that can occur in the fascial body. In a way, the joints can change shape.

For this process to begin, one needs to practice regularly, several times a week, for one or two years. My first teacher, Dan Fanthorpe, used to tell me that students collect the low-hanging fruit of their practice in the first year or two, and then come up against more entrenched characteristics of the body. This is very often the case, the journey of the first couple of years of practice is frequently a string of achievements. At some point, progress can seem to slow as the limit of tougher tissue is reached[51].

Nonetheless, people who continue to practice beyond this point progress indefinitely. I have seen people who cannot touch their toes go on to put their legs behind their head, I have seen people with planks of wood for spines progress to smooth and confident back-bends. I have witnessed and experienced all kinds of amazing transformations, and the common ingredient in 100% of cases is the practice of a set sequence of poses, several times per week, over a few years.

You can experience this yourself if you make that commitment. It requires you to struggle in a sense, at least for a while. You must reconcile your feelings of despair in the face of inability to succeed quickly. It requires you to trust that you are empowered to modify your physical existence. That trust grows as you receive gradual glimpses of ease, accomplishments you weren't expecting, and realisations that you have changed. Along the way this alters your psychology profoundly: patience and quiet, focused determination sprouts.

When a long-sought physical pose is eventually accomplished, it's a surreal moment, and something of an anti-climax a lot of the time. You can finally do the pose! But could it have been achieved without all the frustration? What you gain on a subtle level along the way over those couple of years is a far greater reward, and you smile in that way the Buddha smiles — wry and knowing, peaceful and content.

---

[51] Sharath mentioned too that only after the second year of practice do students start to realise the less physical aspects of practice, more clarity, and in-depth understanding.

I remember learning to do deeper backbends. My teacher Dan was encouraging me to deepen the stretch in the classic wheel pose — *ūrdhva dhanurāsana*. It was very difficult. It's worth noting that before I started doing *yoga*, I had a reasonable level of flexibility. I could sort-of barely do a wheel, and I could touch my toes with straight legs.

Dan would encourage me to walk my hands closer to my feet during the wheel poses and I always gave it a good go. In a Mysore style class, this sort of progress is possible in a safe way — the student has as much time as they like to check how their body is feeling, to establish the right attitude, and to experiences ups and downs.

After a lot of frustration and one memorable bump on the head, I was finally able to stand up and drop back from wheel by myself. Yet he still encouraged me to create an even deeper back-bend by walking the hands in, each practice. I recall one day after this, laying on the ground with a familiar dull ache in my back, the kind that subsides after a few minutes. I thought to myself "Am I going to regret this in a few years? Am I being irresponsible?".

More time passed and one day it dawned on me out of the blue, "Hey I used to feel pain here, but not anymore. I don't even need to warm-up to do this pose." These bodily modifications occur so gradually that you often don't experience them as a specific moment of success, you just realise one day that you're different. A regular practice combined with consistent and moderate effort yields incredible things.

Modern pain research reveals that sensations of painful tightness often do not correlate with actual physical restriction or injury. That is, a limb or joint could move further if it weren't for the pain generated within the brain that does not need to be there. We assume that feelings of pain exist when a physical injury is imminent or present, but quite often they serve no physically protective purpose.

Understanding for yourself how things ought to feel is a beautiful journey. On the journey we can gain advice from teachers and professional bodyworkers, but ultimately it is **you** that creates and experiences your physical environment.

One of my favourite photos, shown here, was taken at sunrise at Newcastle Beach with no warmup; I had not practiced at all that morning. This is the morning when I realised that where there was once pain and fear, there now exists comfort.

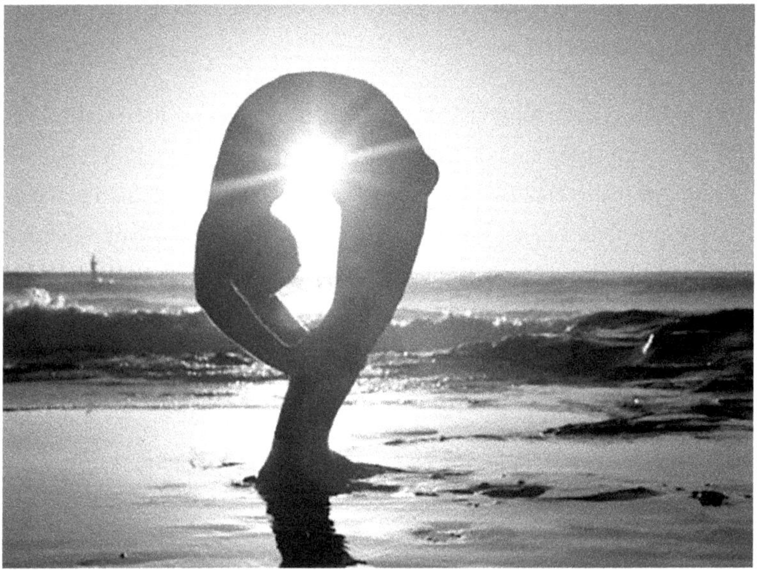

Photo credit: Cat Mead

The virtues of repetition

Ashtanga Vinyasa Yoga is a conditioning process. The student is repeatedly asked to try to do something great — a pose involving stretching and strengthening and deep breathing — with as much smoothness as possible. The student desires to be able to do this and thus feels some self-generated excitement. The student attempts it potentially hundreds of times. Each time, they dissolve and resolve the very meaning of words such as "failure" and "success".

Each time this action is carried out, the unconscious mind is aware of what has happened, and a story unfolds. It is a non-verbal story of intention and persistence. If it were to be verbalised it might sound like: "I made an effort, I put effort into improving myself. I do it every morning and I will keep doing it. I am a person who keeps moving in the direction of positive growth, even when success is not instant."

Students spend 60-90 minutes a day continuously training their minds in this way. This is referred to in Sanskrit as *bhāvana*. A pleasant side-effect of the mental conditioning is oxygenation of the physical system, development of hormonal balance, stretching open the ribs, drawing the shoulders back, making the legs and spine long and strong.

Students naturally stand up taller in life, they are more physically comfortable and they look healthy and confident. Behaviours become more positive — without thinking about it. Someone who stands tall and looks comfortable and behaves positively comes across as trustworthy and successful, and their life tends to exhibit these qualities.

The repetitive nature of this system ensures that the student experiences consistent and gradual improvement, with the most positive reinforcement gained through postures that take the longest to accomplish. This is in contrast to led classes, where there is an emphasis on variety as well as a limited amount of time and many opportunities to tune out or gloss over poses that would otherwise be of great assistance.

A Mysore style practice is an opportunity to create a feeling of loving, positive expectation, and in doing so move up the spiritual mountain while bringing the physical element along for the ride. Instead of escaping and leaving the world behind, separating or distracting, everything is brought along with you in a bold act of integration. This style of practice asks us to show patience and persistence, and in doing so we gain levitation-like physical skills.

Prāṇāyāma during āsana

Prāṇāyāma is the science of breath and considered the aspect of practice that one should tackle after setting up fundamental bodily health through āsana. An incredible feature of Ashtanga Vinyasa Yoga is that it contains a miniature *prāṇāyāma* practice within it.

Take for example the *prāṇāyāma* technique called *bhastrikā*. This is the most powerful technique in the *prāṇāyāma* toolkit, and that the soil must adequately prepared before unleashing its powerful waves of energy[52]. Conveniently, the soil is being prepared all throughout āsana practice.

This particular *prāṇāyāma* technique is referred to as "thoracic bellowing" and can be explored during *sūrya namaskāra*. Step one of *sūrya namaskāra* involves a large intake of air, wild expansion of the frontline of the body, stretching the pericardium, a minor internal breath hold, and mental concentration on the crown of the head. Step two is a complete exhalation during a forward fold, a contraction of abdominal muscles — or more precisely an engagement of the bandhas.

Similarly, the *prāṇāyāma* technique called *kumbhaka* (suspension of breathing) can be included in *āsana* practice. This is something that is not often discussed in the Ashtanga Vinyasa Yoga canon. I learned it from my original teacher, Dan Fanthorpe, and from Śrīvatsa Ramaswami, one of Krishnamacharya's last students. Krishnamacharya himself included specific instructions in his book Yoga Makaranda.

---

[52] Maehle. G., *Pranayama: The Breath of Yoga* (Crabbes Creek: Kaivalya Publications 2014)

For example:

1. *ekam* inhale – raise arms – internal *kumbhaka*
2. *dvi* exhale – bend forward – external *kumbhaka*
3. *trīṇi* inhale – lift your chest – internal *kumbhaka*
4. *catvāri* exhale – jump back, lower down – external *kumbhaka*
5. *pañca* inhale – open chest, extend spine – internal *kumbhaka*
6. *ṣaṭ* exhale – tuck the chin, lift hips – free breathing five times
7. *sapta* inhale – jump to hands open chest – internal *kumbhaka*
8. *aṣṭa* exhale – tuck the chin and fold – external *kumbhaka*
9. *nava* inhale – raise arms – internal *kumbhaka*
10. *daśa* exhale – *samasthiti*

A high degree of strength and flexibility in the nervous system and bodily organs is required for *prāṇāyāma* to be successful, and it makes sense to get a head-start on this training during *āsana*. A simple example would be to implement *kumbhaka* in each of the nine steps in *sūrya namaskāra*, alternating between internal and external retention. From the initial stance of *samasthiti*, inhale and take the arms up over the head and then hold the breath in for a moment, before exhaling as you bend down to the floor, and so forth.

Effective implementation of *kumbhaka* requires training of the *bandha*, which is emphasised in the Ashtanga Vinyasa Yoga system and explained very well by popular authors. It means muscular activation around specific joints or areas of the body, you can create a shoulder or knee *bandha*, for example. The idea is to engage joint complexes in an efficient and safe fashion when performing poses or transitions.

The three most famous *bandha* are called *jalandhara*, *uḍḍīyana*, and *mūla*. In serious *prāṇāyāma*, the inhale and exhale portion of the breath is extended a great deal, as is the duration of holding the breath. To acquire the goal is challenging — we are talking about being able to stretch a single breath out to be one or two minutes long.

The intelligence of Ashtanga Vinyasa Yoga lies here, in the blending of various techniques into the physical *āsana* practice, in particular the movements of the sun salutations.

Breath retention expands the present moment

Sooner or later, a daily seated *prāṇāyāma* practice is introduced to students' daily routine. Focusing on extending the ingoing and outgoing breath as well as the length of breath retention, measured using a metronome, will result in some profound transformations.

The normal experience of thoughts occurring is that you notice a thought suddenly arise, and then you do something with it, you follow or resolve it in some way. When intense *prāṇāyāma* bloomed for me, I increasingly noticed geometries in consciousness. It was quite uncanny.

I realised that I had accrued a new kind of feeling of elevation and quietness. It had come so gradually I hadn't noticed it was there. What sparked my awareness of it was a peculiar sensation — I noticed that thoughts seemed to occur in the distance, away from me. There was now a proximal aspect to thought. There was a feeling of ease, and the sensing of unmanifest thoughts, and the choice to allow them to come closer or to wave them away.

Rather than have an irritation or anxiety pop up, and then either let it run its course or grapple with it using an intellectual strategy, I could feel the thought in proximity to me, in the distance, only slightly existing. Proto-thoughts would simply raise their hand as an invitation, rather than landing in the brain like a projectile. I realised that I felt a sense of dissociated awareness, and it felt good — a different kind of "good".

Rather than having sensations in my mind of a gratifying nature, the usual definition of pleasure, I had a sense of quiescent-euphoria, like viewing a terrain from up high. A sense of pure free will, of being abundant with options, and of having no compulsion or requirement to select anything unless and until I chose.

This is what is meant by the spiritual notions of peace and non-attachment. It's not an escape or an anaesthetisation. Rather, it's a viewpoint that allows you to be more attentive, sensitive, and careful. You care for your thoughts as children or pets, little critters on the fields interacting with each other, with their own traits and tendencies. When children throw a tantrum, a competent parent does not join the tantrum but allows it to exist, guides it and lets it run its course with as little impact as possible. In this way, we become supervisors and guides.

The state of meditation can occur any time

"I've tried meditating, but I can't". This is a comment I frequently hear from people. A popular understanding is that meditation is as an emptying of the mind — an impossible and unnecessary task.

Meditation is an acceptance of more of the mind in varied and subtle ways. Remember too, that this is an English word with a Latin root. At some point in modern history, someone made an equivalency between this word and the Sanskrit term *dhyāna*, and it has been further linked with a diverse range of topics from many modern and ancient teachings. It is preferable to step away from modern words and their associations.

What we actually seek in meditation is a recognition of the other, less obvious aspects of the Self and how they relate to one another. This recognition appears with greater frequency and intensity over time. This is the real definition of a meditative state.

The natural development of a body that is fit and strong and capable, with a large lung capacity and an easy state of calm repose — all of this comes with *yoga*. Even greater is the attainment and sustenance of a poised state where hard distinctions between forms vanish.

Just as a perfectly still lake looks very different to one with ripples and stirring activity, so too is the special clarity of a meditative mind. This is far more profound than stress-relief. The mind becomes a mirror, something that can reveal images far outside its scope. A lake is a body of water, particles of hydrogen and oxygen interspersed with water-dwelling creatures, buffeted by wind and held together with gravity.

It is a complex entity, with many actions of many kinds occurring constantly within. When the surface is completely stilled, however, a lake can reflect the image of anything that exists: a nearby tree, mountains, or a galaxy of stars. When perfectly still, ordinary functions are transcended without being disowned. In this quiescent and upwards gazing state called *unmanī*, information alien to itself can exist upon it.

Your mind is that lake, normally occupied with many fragments and actions. If someone tells you that your mind can display rich information from outside itself on a galactic scale simply by becoming perfectly still, do you believe them? This is called "identification", to clearly display something on consciousness, to mirror an object in the mind. It is a major focus of the Yoga Sūtras of Patañjali[53].

The term *kevala kumbhaka* refers to the spontaneous emergence of the state of meditative absorption. It is the delightful fruit of your practice, your *sādhana*. Instances sprout in the same way as a blooming garden that we have cultivated. We take care of the soil and the water, and then tend to the healthy development of the plants, watching them grow and keeping an eye on the general direction of the shoots.

So too do we keep watching the whole organism of our *yoga* practice. We trust that the fruits will bloom and we have a good idea where and when we will see them, but there is still a mysterious timing at play. We awake each morning and look to see what has ripened overnight, what surprises are ready for us to imbibe.

Rhythm and repetition

Mysore style practice involves rhythm and repetition to keep the body and the brain occupied, lest the mind-body complex fall asleep or become restless and noisy. When you have learned a sequence of postures and can practice them by yourself, quietly, you drop into a calm state very quickly.

---

[53] Also note the same analogy in Aṣṭāvakra Gītā 18.60

You come in and out of it to be sure; distraction still occurs, but in smaller quantities. There is an exponential benefit, an accelerated reward for a consistent and earnest approach.

For many people, entering a state where the mind is not either hyperactive or asleep is almost never experienced. However, if you can actively induce this for consecutive moments on a regular basis, you will experience a snowball effect. Sometimes it's called the "flow state" and it occurs with activities that are fully engaging of one's attention.

We seek a kind of trance state where the coarse physicality is being employed in a repetitive way. The routine of *sūrya namaskāra*, up-dog followed by down-dog, over and over again for an hour or more, opens a channel and allows the effulgence in and then it stays with you for the rest of the day. Ashtanga Vinyasa Yoga is an efficient and safe way to do this, and what it requires is a consistent practice, preferably in the mornings, preferably most days of the week.

Every morning a little more opening, and then, all day we experience integration in the world in our regular life. Each day is an assimilation of self-generated higher energy. It is you that does the work; it is you that feels everything. Often only a nominal amount of instruction is required when we pursue this course; we mostly require simple supervision and an occasional sounding board.

Practicing *yoga* in a Mysore style setting, rather than a led class format, clearly shares interoception-enhancing qualities with musicianship and dance. All three are activities performed individually while also in a group. They all require personal responsibility and commitment to earnest effort, finesse, fine-tuned inner awareness, and all are usually practiced in concert with a group. In this way, each class is a song of harmonious melodies and tempos.

In fact, this opening up is so gradual that it is barely noticed, and this is the way it ought to be. Ask a long-term student if they have felt their "central channel" open and the "nectar of immortality" flow and they may well look at you like you're crazy. But their lives show the traits of a person who has become more potent and decisive, and more capable of compassion to all, with a minimum of fuss.

The state of absorption slows down time

There is a process in *yoga* referred to as *laya*, whereby fragmented pieces of content in consciousness merge into one coherent form. During *laya*, the witness moves up the metaphorical mountain so that the pieces can all be viewed at the same time. It is translated in English as absorption or blending, and we will see that Mysore style classes encourage this process to occur.

When one's view of content is blended, the experience of time changes. In the usual chattering mental mode, the coarse mind steps from piece to piece in a repetitive act of linear deliberation. This is the mundane waking state in which there is a need for many thought-steps.

At the conclusion of the process the pieces are merged and no steps are required. Even the word "conclusion" becomes redundant. There is no movement through space. All is apprehended in one instant that contains all of time. There is one large moment instead of many small moments. Ornate concepts can be held in the mind and float on the screen of consciousness. View them from various angles without talking to yourself.

The absorptive state is made possible with *pratyāhāra*, the total inward turning of attention to the extent that physical senses are no longer employed. Externalised sense perception switches to internalised. BNS Iyengar says that inward turning of attention reveals "inner words and intuition."

You don't hear or see things around you as you are "in the zone". You are pushing up against the threshold of dream consciousness. When you do emerge, it feels a bit like waking up or coming out of a trance, and when you check the clock, more apparent time has flown by than you thought.

There are other things that occur in conscious experience when the border of deep imagination and the waking state is explored, such as subtle inner sounds. These sounds are called *nāda* in Sanskrit, and concentration on them is a most potent form of meditation, one that is prescribed in the opening parts of Yoga Tārāvalī. You may not notice, but at the point of falling asleep, high pitched sounds are present. They occur moments before you fall asleep and are usually forgotten. With the exploration of absorptive states, these and other curious phenomena are noticed.

We know that sleeping dreams seem like long adventures and yet occur in a very short period of ordinary physical time. You might experience two hours of activity in a dream and yet only a few minutes of physical time have passed. How efficient! Imagine if this could be accessed at will; work could be done on a level far more malleable and unconstrained, rather than needing to spell everything out in discrete physical steps.

Yoga provides extensive methods of inducing states of *laya*, absorption. The aim is to momentarily dissociate the witnessing self from the ordinary mental operations, to break the addiction to thinking and talking and mechanical action. Ordinarily, it is common to forget that we can gain a higher perspective and orchestrate our lives better. *Yoga* prescribes an array of physical and mental techniques that act as a circuit breaker, something akin to stepping up to a lookout and — suddenly struck — to gaze breathlessly across incredible landscapes.

One could be mistaken for thinking these states of effulgence and swooning trances are the final aims of the practice, so delightful they are. But they are merely tools and signposts on the journey to reaching this higher consciousness. How wonderful that in addition to their adaptive functions, they are also joyous and ecstatic in themselves. It's almost as though we evolved to seek them out.

To avoid growth by fixating on tiny steps and inner ruminations takes effort, and it ages us. The sunlight of our higher consciousness is always there, immense, ready for us to soak and blossom. You can be aware of your power, perceive opportunities, and choose what to invoke.

The only limits are beliefs, assumptions, and suppressed passion and curiosity. So, let your rigidity dissolve, and set up new frameworks in the spirit of playfulness and experimentation. It is up to the individual to seek and align consciously with ideas that they find personally exciting.

There is also even psychological research on the topic of awe as something that seems to foster prosocial behaviour that shifts attention to a bigger picture beyond the concerns of the individual[54].

Every individual can live a life of unmitigated joy; any mitigation that exists currently is optional. There's nothing you need to do to earn bliss and free will; you already deserve it and always have. Just find the positive in every single thing, in every single moment, until it becomes your default automatic program. It is a magnetic attraction to the upside.

---

[54] Piff et al., "Awe, the Small Self, and Prosocial Behavior," Journal of Personality and Social Psychology, Vol. 108, 2015

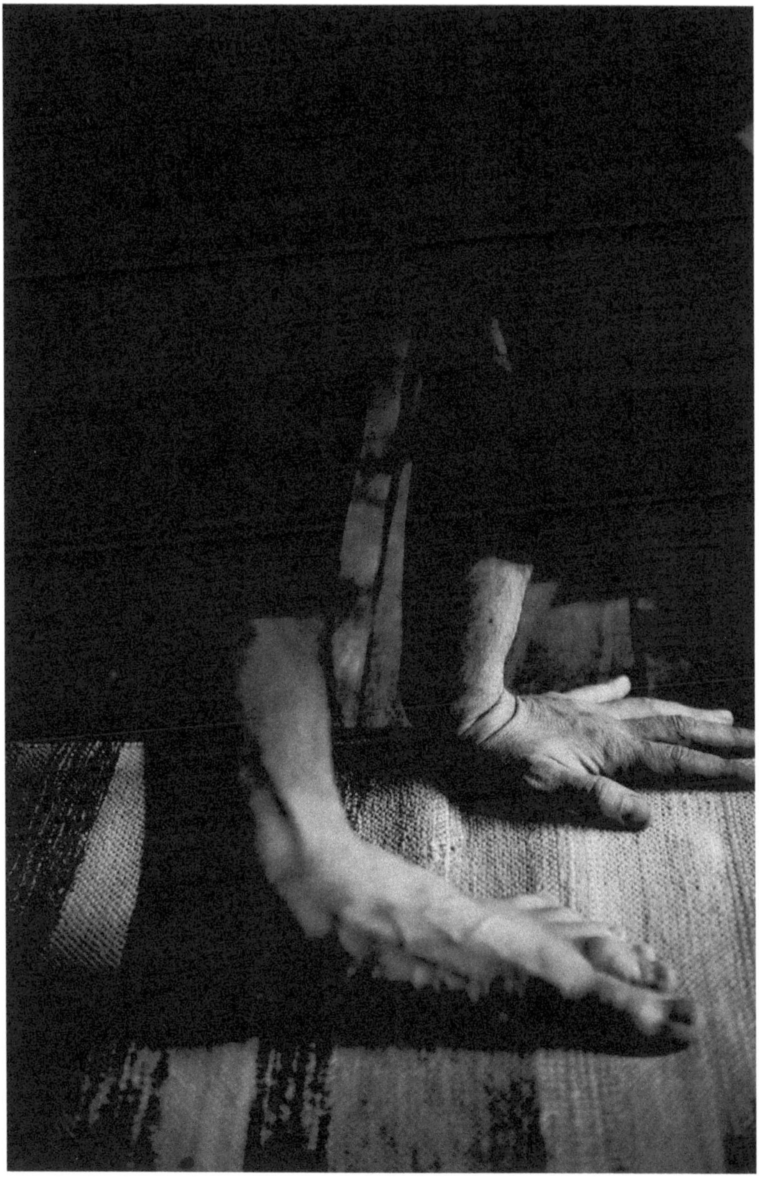

Photo credit: Kate Binnie

5

THE UPDRAFT

The intermediate series is infamous

Over the time a student learns the primary series, many fundamental assumptions about what is possible are rewritten, and this has direct and profound consequences for the personality and mental state. On the physical level, the lower back and hips are stretched and mobilised, and the upper body and core are strengthened.

The purpose of the second, or intermediate, series of Ashtanga Vinyasa Yoga is to enjoy the body's newfound capacity to move and float. This next series of postures carves new channels in the mind-body complex. There are forward and backward bends included in more equal proportions as compared to the primary series, which is focused on forward bends.

It could certainly be said that the intermediate series is the most balanced one, and is best to be practiced all through a human life.

As you proceed through the series you continue to experience openings in the body and fewer restrictive beliefs; you thought that bending over backwards like that would kill you. But it didn't — now it feels good.

So, you begin to seek that kind of challenge; you understand that thrill and excitement is a sign of something bigger on the horizon. Blossoming and flowering occurs — the brightest whites radiate, milky moons reflect, ecstatic experiences of dissociation await.

The two-phase repetitive cycle of spirituality continues to play out. Deep and intensely introspective forward folds morph into even deeper leg-behind-the-head poses. Then we switch for the sake of expansion, delving into incredible backbends, indicating trust and openness. We express gratitude for the gift of a material body and life.

I remember in my days in Gokulam, Mysore, hanging out at a café with other students. One of them informed me that, when performed correctly, *yoga* is not supposed to deliver you a standard "exercise high". This was totally new information to me, having initially learned a group-fitness style of class. Here I was parading around the streets doing chin-ups on street signs and drinking caffeine energy drinks in the waiting room before practice. I was such a rascal! In the same trip I remember busting out a *kapotāsana* on a café lounge during breakfast to show off.

It's easy to see how people could get stuck on a cycle of excessive sympathetic nervous system activation doing gym classes, which they then need to fix using *yin* classes where poses are held for 5-10 minutes, de-escalating the nervous system and providing a more relaxed experience of stretching — a somewhat bipolar situation[55]. In Mysore style classes you learn about your own personal middle path.

---

[55] Far be it for me to judge: during those India visits, practicing amongst the world's best, this same rascal established an ibuprofen-on-an-empty-stomach pre-practice performance enhancement regime, in addition to the caffeine, that lasted a few years until my stomach gave clear indications of distress. I was very liberal with drugs those days; it is fortunate that I did not find any opium dens in the city!

Peak performance

In many ways, *yoga* is the science of peak performance. We learn how to adjust our nervous system to suit the task at hand, to switch between *rajas* or arousal (sympathetic nervous system activation), and *tamas* or relaxation (parasympathetic nervous system activation).

When we need to rise to a challenge, our *yoga* training allows the body-brain complex to quickly activate hormones and neurological circuits that help us perform the task in a skilled and efficient way. When we need to regenerate or access creative ideation, we can do so more quickly and deeply. Less time is spent trying to relax or get to sleep, and more time is spent in the most desired states of rest or visualisation. For each, there are specific techniques that can be employed as needed, but also note that the medium-term practice of *yoga* automatically makes this process smoother.

You begin to realise that you are both rising to challenges and coming to rest with less friction and delay. You come to notice that you are flowing through peaks of arousal and valleys of relaxation far more easily than before, and you notice the same in others who practice.

This idea of optimal performance, being nimble and efficient, is an excellent hook to entice modern folk to invest in a consistent *yoga* practice. Our culture highly values being entrepreneurial and productive, so a legal method for people to boost their intelligence and energy without inducing insomnia is attractive.

The best way to improve functional performance for many people is to help them relax better at night — and to give them permission to seek small doses of unstructured creative rest during the day. Rather than plough headlong in only one direction, we want the ability to pause, and in Mysore style classes permission is granted to take pauses. It becomes obvious to students that setting their own pace during strenuous activity actually increases efficiency and pleasure. In a gym class — *yoga* or otherwise — resting means having to sit out and miss part of the class.

In a Mysore style class, it is not unusual to see a legitimate athlete perform complex and impressive feats, sweating and exerting, and to then lay down for 1-2 minutes, calming themselves. After a short rest, they bounce up again and proceed through the next poses in their sequence. They have not missed any poses; they are simply learning to regulate their effort in harmony with the circumstances in that moment.

From the point of calm personal power, we can optimise our path. How wonderful it is for our culture when we can demonstrate to others a merging of worldly success with states of ease, joy, and integrity.

Nature is habitual

The ordinary physical experience consists of polarities, in Sanskrit the word is *dvandva*. It refers to pairs of opposites, particularly taking the form of duels, dilemmas, quarrels, contests, and complications. It is witnessed in the world as compulsive, mechanical, or unthinking attractions and aversions. The process of *yoga* is to explore these biases and beliefs, especially those that have are so ingrained as to be almost invisible, in as many forms and domains as possible. The objective is to then **consciously** set them according to our higher and inspired wishes.

Sometimes habits and tendencies are framed as insurmountable obstacles, but this need not be the case, and *yoga* provides tools to re-establish free-will. Every time this is done, the influence of prior events is superseded. The collection of habits we possess is referred to as our *karma*, and by implementing free-will like this we transcend our *karma*. We acknowledge paradox and duality, in order to make fresh and truthful decisions.

The word *karma* is a tricky one as it tends to bring up ideas from modern religion, popular misconceptions, and superstition. The root of the word, *kṛ*, means "to act", and it is extended in this case to mean a cluster of actions linked together by a chain of causation. Each action has a varying degree of conscious selection, unconscious bias or external influence attached to it. There can be long or short chains of actions, as well as recurring ones or easily changeable ones.

A *karmic* tendency is a cluster of the modes of nature. There are three modes of nature, called *guṇa*-s. The term *rajas* denotes passion or striving, *tamas* is lack or passivity, and *sattva* indicates an harmonious and neutral b~~lend of the two~~. neither one nor the other

On the atomic scale the interaction of *rajas* and *tamas* is reflected in the flow of electricity, as electrons move from atoms with an abundance of electrons to atoms with a scarcity of electrons. On the cosmic scale we see that planetary bodies will possess the quality of *rajas* or *tamas* with respect to their propensity to draw objects into their gravitational field, or to be drawn into one themselves.

This is a useful model on the human psychological scale as well. See the example below for a simple *karmic* cluster, a habit that one might have, a combination of attraction, aversion, and choice:

"When I sense an opportunity for intellectual sparring (*tamas* — a space devoid of conflict), I choose to provoke (*rajas* — create conflict in the space). I derive a sense of enjoyment and satisfaction from this particular kind of interplay (*sattva* — the blending of opposites)."

With *yoga* we expose **unconscious** attractions and aversions, habits and programs, and we shine the light of consciousness upon them so they are visible and can be reviewed. These programs play out so quickly that they can be difficult to spot. Behaviour seems to occur instantly; biases are handed down to us and only sometimes noticed or questioned.

We use tools of *yoga* to detach from tendencies. We do this, most fundamentally, by actively **imagining** or **acting out** a tendency that is the opposite to our current position.

Try to imagine or mimic an opposing view, something you disagree with, until it is actually felt and agreed with conviction. This is an important practice, mentally and physically. This is a fusion of opposites — paradoxical and liberating.

We must all be willing and able to drop, for a moment, long held beliefs and then pick up and hold sincerely the opposite belief. If your original view is true and useful, it will come back as a freshly selected conscious preference rather than an automatic bias. You will also have new information from your empathetic exploration.

Training your mind like this will present ease or difficulty depending on your personal traits. There will be many tendencies that seem rigid and inflexible. Effortlessly empathising with the opposite view may not be possible right away, but if we understand the logic of the process, we can look at techniques to encourage some movement.

This search for knowing and understanding, resulting in peace, is a native human drive. To have both sides of the story, to be balanced, is another example of *sattva*, the harmonious collaboration of opposites.

So innate is this drive that, funnily enough, the approach of the dispassionate scientist and the approach of stereotypically nurturing and "emotional" people can be equalised. When a scientist discovers a blind spot or bias, they are glad to have found it and they seek to learn about it. When a nurturing person discovers their inability to grasp the point of view of another, they seek to empathise and understand. Both run on the same natural drive, expressed differently.

Become a natural back-bender

An obvious and visceral way to look at our biases is by working with the physical body. Usually, a person will create a body that is more comfortable either forward-folding or back-bending, to some degree.

The intermediate series of Ashtanga Vinyasa Yoga helps to neutralise this by bending deeply in each direction — forwards and backwards — so frequently that any bias is gradually erased and both options become equally available. This is one of the most intense procedures that we can implement on ourselves.

Steeped in lore, this series of postures has been known to invoke signs of lunacy in people. Students speak of insomnia and a shaking of foundations. The need for the grounding work of the primary series, and a teacher and community, is thus reinforced.

Through exploring deeply these positive and negative positions, we purify our mind and body. Points of attachment are brought to the surface, heat and agitation are shaken off as a by-product, and the path is cleared for the ultimate conversion into a being who acts through conscious selection.

The knots we find in our mind are our judgements, assumptions, and fixed positions. They colour our experience and represent the template from which our reality is generated. They can be cleared out, especially those that have been handed down, those that have been accepted without examination, those which stoke feelings of fear, lack, and other neurotic thoughts associated with the survival instinct.

Smoothing out knots in your energy channels is like removing kinks from a blocked garden hose. A gradual approach is usually a good idea — simply turning the tap on more and increasing the water pressure might be enough to free it up, but might also be uncomfortable or ineffective, even to the point of arousing violent effects.

Ashtanga Vinyasa Yoga, and especially the intermediate series, is used to gradually work loose these obstacles. During practice we discover rigidities and then we rejoice in them, validate and study them. In time, empathy is fully developed in that part of the body, healing occurs, and we become able to exercise a fuller range of movement and possibility.

In this way, we find practical equanimity and are empowered to select. Obtaining a real grasp on this is important. The intention of science and spirituality is the same — to increase knowledge and thus free will.

Uniformity pervades

Imagine if you could see, for example, a broader band of the visible light spectrum. If the eyes of a human were configured to see microwave radiation, our understanding of the world would be very different. Many beliefs and assumptions in human culture are contingent on a very narrow way of viewing the world, and they would break down with greater sensory bandwidth.

It is a non-controversial truth that there is very little distinction between the invisible air we breathe and the seemingly solid objects we touch, other than an arbitrary line drawn by the genetically determined boundaries of human sense organs.

Any distinction we perceive between "solid objects" is only due to the very narrow band of data that our five senses detect. Radio waves, wireless signals, and cosmic background radiation is passing through your body, right now, as though you barely exist.

With this somewhat unsettling information, humankind searches for order, and it frequently looks to the seemingly empty space pervading the material world. There is a field of electromagnetic activity, swirling and moving, invisible to human eyes. Similarly, there is a field upon which, or from which, all matter emerges — a universal substrate.

To understand this is a key pursuit of science and spirituality alike. Through history, it has been pointed at using ideas like the aetheric medium that is more subtle than light and exists beyond the sphere where classical physical laws function. Refer to notions of panpsychism where some mind-like aspect pervades all of the material world. More recently, quantum fields that are more fundamental than particles, and the unified field consisting of physical and virtual fields.

The modern academic approach of naming an object and then studying it as though it is separate from the person studying it is the mode of learning employed by the linear intellect. The more direct approach discussed by *yoga* is to silently **identify** with an object. The word identify is used in a very careful way — the Sanskrit term is *saṃyama*, which means "to bind consciousness to an object".

When you perform *saṃyama* on an object — when you identify with it — you mirror the object in your consciousness to the extent that it exists perfectly accurately within you, and you thus know it by direct perception. The object becomes intimately familiar. It is called non-dual knowledge.

Scientific and spiritual investigation both point to the same obvious requirement that there is something from which tangible matter springs. Arguing about what to call this could consume lifetimes.

The Indians refer to it using different terms depending on the era and school of knowledge that you look at. It is commonly known as *brahman* or *ākāśa*, and *yoga* provides methods of identifying with and thus learning about this field in various kinds of *saṃyama* and *samādhi*.

Ecstatic surge

As with a slightly kinked garden hose, turning on the tap and allowing a good burst of energy might be all we need to get a move on. If you found a short-cut to rapidly increase the energy in your conscious experience, it would be tempting to use it — perhaps at your peril…

The techniques of the intermediate series represent such a boost. The combination of deep forward and backward bends stimulates the release of substances in the body that assist in transcending existing patterns.

Cerebrospinal fluid (CSF) is an ultrafiltrate of plasma that moves around the spine and into spaces in the brain, in dynamic relationship with our posture, heartbeat and breath. It provides nutrients (proteins, hormones, and sugar), waste removal, and shock absorbing physical protection[56]. It flows into the third ventricle of the brain and it touches the pineal gland.

[56] Spector R, Robert Snodgrass S, Johanson CE, "A balanced view of the cerebrospinal fluid composition and functions: Focus on adult humans," Exp Neurol. 2015 Nov

It also contains dimethyltryptamine (DMT)[57], which is a potent psychedelic drug that can be used to burst through limited belief systems that are commonly taught to us as children. Anecdotally it aligns with the famous ambrosial nectar known as *amṛta* which has a distinctly salty-sweet taste, and the smooth onset of psychedelia can be noticed when it is ingested. Adults generate around 500mL of CSF per day, and it is constantly being secreted and recirculated. A lack of mobility has been associated with aging and neurodegenerative disease[58].

It has been claimed that *prāṇāyāma* and *yoga āsana* (and the intermediate series in particular) increases mobility of cerebrospinal fluid[59] and its reabsorption. Techniques of *haṭha yoga* such as *khecarī mudrā* also directly encourage this to occur. Other avenues available include fasting, *bhastrikā*, *kumbhaka*, and *yoga nidrā.*

There is support in modern studies for the idea that the roof of the mouth and its manipulation with the tongue, assisted by the tensing and suction effects of the *bandha*, is a key to psychedelic ecstasies and access to the *ājñā cakra* through the fabled pineal gland. It has been noted that the pineal gland is formed in the foetus from tissue of the roof of the mouth and later moves to its position in the ventricle of the brain, near the blood-brain barrier, where it may be stimulated.

In *śloka* 6-7 of Yoga Tārāvalī it is explained that "the beautiful serpentine form of *kuṇḍalinī* arises from her dormant state by means of the powerfully arousing action bending and contortion of the physical body, causing an overflow of nectar to stream". The intermediate series of Ashtanga Vinyasa Yoga, practiced in a Mysore style setting, also offers a gradual, safe, and fun way to achieve these results.

---

[57] M.A.Geyer, D.E.Nichols, F.X. Vollenweider, "Serotonin-Related Psychedelic Drugs", Reference Module in Neuroscience and Biobehavioral Psychology 2017

[58] L Sakka, G Coll, J Chazal, "Anatomy and physiology of cerebrospinal fluid," European Annals of Otorhinolaryngology, Head and Neck Diseases, Vol. 128, Issue 6, Dec 2011

[59] Delaidelli and Moiraghi, "Respiration: A New Mechanism for CSF Circulation?" Journal of Neuroscience, 26 Jul 2017

Not much of this has been formally studied in clinical settings in the West, but you can perform the experiments yourself and compare your findings to the testimony of ancient *yoga* texts. Whatever the technical mechanism, the effect of these practices is most certainly replicable, and within Mysore style classes experiments can be undertaken safely.

Once a student has access to techniques that allow for removal of constrictions and biases, the question remains of what to do next. A clear mind, greater sense of free will, and transcendence of former attractions and aversions gives space for creative imagination and inspired action.

Hold a clear vision in the mind with a combination of intention, concentration, aspiration, trust, and surrender. Let it to reside there simultaneously as we operate in the world. Allow the journey towards the desired outcomes to be rendered before our eyes, in real-time, in a creative and ecstatic manner.

When the vision is illumined and there is a curious and whimsical attitude, the simplest acts take on new meaning. Even breathing becomes sanctified. We send out an arrow in the direction of our vision, we cast a net with our senses, and then watch as the net expands and draws in possibilities. Any stray impulses to act in ways that are out of alignment with the vision fall away as we wait for positive and harmonious options to appear. As this habit develops, your actions become automatically purely positive. If you can't find a positive option in consciousness, then wait until your imagination generates something. If it feels fake or forced, that is okay — it will get much easier with practice.

In the real world of competing demands and impulsivity and distraction, the buck stops with action. No matter the mixed-up contents of the mind and the pull of emotions, with action we have control and we ultimately set up our reality using this tool. You create the world.

Each of your actions has multitudinous effects, subtle and obvious. You induce and attract the world with your actions. Create a framework in your imagination, set up the future blueprint and then, crucially, act in this direction. Build an intention in your imagination, and then initiate a cascade of events with your action. When you move in this direction, your perspective expands. You see more order in what seemed like chaos, more causes of events, more ingredients that comprise phenomena.

As we move towards the ineffable, naturally, poetry comes to the fore. The supreme view is of the radiance of creation, the white light that contains all colours. You could reflect the personality of *bhagavan* as it revealed though chapter ten of Bhagavad Gītā. Śaṅkara uses beautiful language all through Saundarya Laharī in devotion to the lotus feet of the goddess *tripurasundarī* — the inference is that what to the lower mind is the ceiling, is merely the floor of the higher mind.

Symbology like this is a necessary part of pointing the mind towards higher ideas. It is all too obvious that there is a tendency for things to go down, a principle of gravity in the mind as it were. Inspiration seems to be interrupted by "grim reality" at some stage. But this entropic tendency is temporary and reversable, and symbols can be used to remind us to attend to aspects of life beyond linearity and materiality.

Swami Prabhupada explains the need for symbols[60]. It is stated that for those whose consciousness is strongly identified with the physical body, it is most difficult to remember the formless and infinite nature of ultimate reality, and thus they require physical symbols that in turn point to non-physical concepts. Whether this is artwork depicting supernatural avatars, or equations depicting quantum entanglement, is up to you and your inclinations.

> *"Recently I was practicing at the beach. It was windy and whilst in śavāsana I could feel the breeze from across the ocean on my face. This sent me on a journey, going through the steps that had created that sensation necessary for the existence of awareness. It led me all the way to the fusion of hydrogen to helium in the centre of the sun which created the energy to warm the air on earth which resulted in the wind. And in that moment, everything was connected, not just the wind and sun, but everything, and I was the sun."*
> *– Mysore student*

---

[60] Swami Prabhupāda, *Bhagavad Gītā As It Is* (India: The Bhaktivedanta Book Trust, 1972) *śloka* 12.5 commentary notes

Tools to realise the higher mind

To go beyond the normal scope of ordinary mentality requires something special, an increase in dimension. Imagine looking at one face of a coin. This is a two-dimensional plane, and only one face can be viewed at a time. To see the whole coin consisting of both faces you'll need three-dimensional awareness. Additionally, to see the coin spin in the air and move along a trajectory, you'll need four dimensions.

The surface layer of mind, the basic dialoguing brain, is concerned with stimulus and response, and it adheres to linear progressions of action and verbalisation. This is the first dimension we seek to tame.

This surface layer of mind is perhaps the most tangible aspect of what makes us human and has been much studied and lauded in modern history. We find this aspect so measurable and comfortable to deal with that the study of it is given scientific names (psychology and neuroscience), upon which are conferred a level of trust.

Over time this focus on the surface mind has resulted in a forgetting of the higher mind that consists of rapid successions of information dense images. It is common to possess a definition, an implicit or explicit assumption that the surface mind is "you". This is what is meant when spiritual teachings refer to the illusory or false self.

The senses observe combinations of measurable material interactions, and often there is a leap made from this observation to the decision that your consciousness and mind are solely born from those interactions. If you find yourself with this assumption, you will need to loosen it a little.

The surface mind has been assigned responsibilities that are beyond its station. It doesn't work far beyond the short-term immediate moments. It doesn't come up with spontaneous and creative ideas. It doesn't do instant and intuitive forecasting, although it can develop tools like computers to assist it. It is the post-hoc rationalisation mind.

Here is another form of the mountaintop metaphor, with a top-down view, called *pañca kośa*:

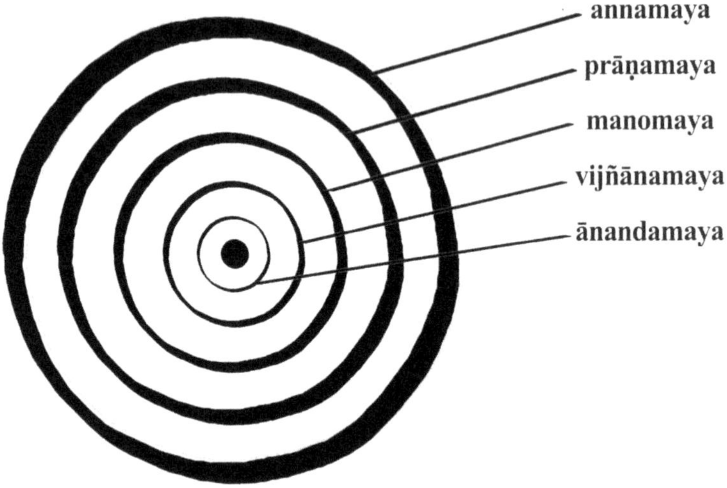

Diagram: The "five sheaths" of being

During *yoga*, we implement the two-stage spiritual process of climbing up (or in) to a higher vantage, combined with relaxing the dialoguing mind and allowing things to be revealed on a plateau. As we go up, it becomes quite clear that there are planes of consciousness more subtle, relatively invisible to the outer rings of the surface mind. These planes work with transcendental concepts like multi-dimensional reality effortlessly.

The sooner we identify this, the better. An exclusively material mindset is not optimal, not by a long shot. We need greater vision. If we restrict ourselves to the assumption that we are flesh-robots compelled by genetic competition, then we are hobbled as a species. There is no need to exclude the rest of reality.

To see more, two things must occur on a regular and rhythmic basis:

1. Recognise and follow the concentrated, aspirational, and eager uplift that everyone possesses in the form of passions and interests that evoke exuberance and joy beyond mere sense indulgence.
2. Calm the brain and body to partake of creative enjoyment, listen to the unfolding of subtle consciousness, and assimilate intuitive messages.

The process of *yoga* is a gradual removal of artifice and suppression that restricts this natural process. Ideas of "sub" and "un" conscious mind fall away, as do notions of higher and lower selves. All is integrated in the Self. We realise the information-dense landscape is always available, although it was previously only seen (and quickly forgotten) in dreams.

The creation of separateness and relationship is the imposition of amnesia, in Sanskrit called *māyā* — forgetting the all-pervading unity.

Bliss is the resolution of polarities

The way that *yoga* delivers such realisations is by disarming filters and judgements that hold the mind to a rigid stance. Attractions and aversions are the mind's attempt to create (an ultimately false) sense of certainty in a world that is fundamentally molten and always changing. This is a coping strategy that we unlearn.

Attractions and aversions, polarities, are not inherently bad; they are a prism through which we interact with three-dimensional reality. They are an operating system that features the experience of otherness, separation, and combinatory play. When we learn how to operate them, we become free, and key to this learning is honouring inner truth, sincerity, and passion, while maintaining calm in the mind.

Our uplift depends on joyful play. The rational mind must come along as well, but passionate exploration is the engine. The idea that bliss and sobriety are mutually exclusive is false — unless you want it to seem so.

Even in the greatest confusion, we know that bliss is preferred over pain. It is the most natural preference. Even if the surface mind has formed the opinion that you do not deserve it, or that it isn't possible to get more than a 50/50 mix of bliss and pain in life, still it is obvious that you would select bliss in any moment it was offered.

Similarly, even if you believe that an absence of pain would somehow make bliss less special, still, only a madman (or perhaps a vengeful sky-god), would design a life that contains compulsory pain.

The highest spiritual bliss is known as *ānanda*. It is always existent and accessible; it is not something generated and it is never missing from your life. We may **notice it** at times of gratification or stimulation and mistakenly conclude that those events created the bliss, but this is not the case. It is fortuitous blends of beliefs and actions that allow the **already existing** and abundant bliss to be felt.

This highest bliss is not an effect in the way that tingling tastebuds is an effect of eating. Bliss is itself an ingredient that exists in all things. It is there always, waiting for us to drop the obscuring artifice, the drudgery of analysis, the lazy cynicism, and identify with it.

Navigate the world of objects with a calm mind that holds effects at bay. Even when faced with slings-and-arrows, we can maintain observation of what pulls us into material obsession, and also what brings us joy and curiosity. Our deepest desires and interests are always there, even if we have pushed them aside — they are the homing beacon.

A mind habituated to honouring its desire for the highest possible constructive adventure in every moment is best poised to live a good life, and to assist others to do the same. Such a state lends itself to realisation of the unity of all diverse elements. Such a state helps us notice that to help an individual always helps the whole.

Note the focus on terms like overtly positive feelings like bliss and excitement. Some schools of spirituality focus on a more modest reduction of suffering, and this is a mistake. Suffering will reduce, but it is only an effect of a greater process. Fixation on effects and symptoms like suffering is a trap of the materialist worldview.

Yoga is not for stress reduction

Let me be clear about the true purpose of *yoga*. It is not for stress reduction, symptom relief and a bland passivity.

An example: look at *prāṇāyāma* for a moment. These days it is often taught as an exercise in mental health first aid. With a sturdy and traditional *prāṇāyāma* practice, you will experience much less stress — that is a legitimate effect — but it is a result of lighting up your positive idealisations so emphatically that fear, guilt, and other neuroses must fall away. Great joy and potency emerge by developing primary biological functions to levels that humans don't ordinarily pursue.

Ashtanga Vinyasa Yoga conducted in a Mysore style setting prepares the student for advanced *prāṇāyāma*. Authentic *prāṇāyāma*, best taught in person by an experienced teacher, consists of elongation of the inhale and the exhale along with extended breath retention. With earnest practice, you come to a recognition that your consciousness extends outwards from your physical body — you gain awareness of the space around your body. You sense thoughts and impressions of yourself and others in your proximity, and you learn to effortlessly either wave them away or permit them to approach you. You feel utter poise and balance.

An athletic *āsana* practice that is centred around the breath, practiced in a Mysore style setting and supplemented by formal *prāṇāyāma* under the supervision of an expert, is how we awaken spiritual knowledge.

High focus

The surface mind is a highly focused tool, like a shovel. It does one thing within a limited scope very well, and repeated use of the tool can move mountains. This mode of existence possesses the fundamental characteristic of forgetfulness. It is hyper-focused on one thing at a time to the exclusion of other things. The surface mind is blinkered — if something is not visible, it does not practically exist. It perceives a subset of reality based on sensory input and defers to memory, testimony, and supposition to cope with what is not visible, such as gravity or oxygen.

Dreams and imagination reflect a very subtle aspect of consciousness and are almost completely outside the scope of the surface mind. The vast majority of what happens in dreams escapes its grip. Things come and go so rapidly they are mostly forgotten before they can be grasped. Yet, without a constant interface with the subtle world, the intellect would be starved, left foraging amongst the mundane.

People tend to believe that dreams are hazy and ambiguous, but they are actually crystal clear. The memory of dreams after you wake is hazy, but the present experience of them is not. Your surface mind forgets them upon waking. Occasionally, you seem to have an especially vivid dream, but it's not that the dream was more vivid. Rather, your surface mind happened to retain it in memory a little better than usual.

Practices of *yoga* thin out the barrier between sleep and waking consciousness and facilitate the revelation that dream activity is much more detailed than ordinary waking perception.

The further up the mountain you travel, the greater the overwhelm for the surface mind. The subtler and higher aspects of mind come to the front and often "knock out" the surface mind, causing you to fall asleep or even physically jolt. When you meditate, you are training yourself to be able to stay awake while this part of your mind is being observed. You are learning to see the dreams without falling into unconsciousness.

This is possible when your curiosity and trust is awakened, and when you put effort into the process. The reality that exists as rapid successions and interactions of vivid imagery is finally noticed by the intellect, which might even agree to take a back seat for a while.

The image-dream landscape is real and comprehensive. It is also happening right now. You are dreaming while you are awake. You are always immersed in detailed and high-resolution streams of concepts and information, but sometimes you pay attention to a spreadsheet or a soccer ball instead. Only when you are asleep — or meditating — does your awareness exclusively point towards that space.

If the assumption is made that dreams and imagination are inconsequential, wistful, and temporary apparitions, then you cut yourself off from most of yourself. This is what *yoga* defines as delusion. If the further mistake is made of appointing the limited and forgetful surface mind, with its attractions and aversions, to the position of controller, then the situation can last innumerable lifetimes.

Yoga is un-filtering

In *yoga* we press the surface mind into service rather than let it consume all our attention. We place it at the feet of the higher by suggesting a new assumption:

The landscape of consciousness, associated with dreams and imagination, which transcends the sense-based operating mode of the surface mind, contains information that is extraordinarily valuable and adaptive. Furthermore, changes and actions made at this higher level of consciousness enable efficient modification of physical circumstances to match our ideals.

To have amnesia lifted is breathtaking — to step up to a lookout or feel the touch of another human. There is much beauty in this game of forgetting and rediscovering. After all, if we could not block out future weight-gain remorse or fear of tooth decay, we would not be able to fully enjoy chocolate.

To experience something as though it was the first time, the thrill of the chase, the sense of accomplishment, is indeed a cherished part of our lives. It is a fun game until we feel bored or confined by it. Our interests elevate, our focus upgrades to more novel targets, until the entire idea of having a specific focus becomes tiresome. At this point the need is felt to break out and expand. We experience the desire to open in some way.

Tools of *yoga* help us unfold at a pace that is exciting and enjoyable. Most common is the eight steps of the "royal path" of *raja yoga*, also known as *aṣṭāṅga yoga*, which culminates in *samādhi*.

In the practice of *samādhi*, we consciously select a principle or sphere of contemplation and practice holding it exclusively in our consciousness. Here again is the two-stage cycle of spiritual practice — alternation between strong focus (*samprajñāta samādhi*) and broad receptivity (*asamprajñāta samādhi*). This is repeated with progressively more subtle topics, until it becomes consistently easy and the viewpoint is elevated and we able to see more. In this practice of bumping up against our limitations, experiences of struggle can be found. But, as with *āsana*, it tends to become easier the more you practice.

Bliss is your guide to the top of the mountain

Blissful tones of elevation and clarification in your individual conscious experience are your guide to the top of the mountain. As you become more familiar with the feeling, as you seek and notice it, you will find that it accompanies and thus indicates **in real-time** the actions in your life that will continue to lift you up, rather than slide you down into states of narrow specificity. Simply put, this is your psychic sense.

This mechanism need not be supernatural or out of reach. The feeling of blissful elevation is your non-verbal trail of bread-crumbs. In any moment you can consider the various actions available to you, and then ask yourself which options evoke this feeling. You swiftly rehearse or project how they would feel, using your imagination. If there are several appealing options, choose the most exciting one. If an option is very exciting but **you** determine that it would do harm or create separation, then rule it out and choose another.

The ability to sense and choose the most interesting path without the distraction of mental chatter or prejudice is the revered discernment called *viveka*. It is momentary by nature, quite serendipitous, and so requires your continued attention. Live your life as a series of exceptional circumstances, each spontaneous and fertile.

There is no escape from the need to be sensitive and fully awake in each moment. You might, for example, suddenly feel like speaking to a stranger you see at the library. This is the only time you have ever felt like doing so — and that is the only time it matters. As you experiment with this, yielding positive results, trust in the process increases and you pay more consistent attention.

The feeling becomes more familiar and natural, and we may notice it in contexts that are not always obviously "positive" — rather more instructive or helpful. You might hear a dog bark in a peculiar way, and it rouses you to take a particular action that is necessary for that moment. It is a sense that carries a gravity, an uncanny importance, an urge for movement. It can be described as the feeling that accompanies the dreams you remember, as well as the feeling of *deja vu*.

This is not a new skill that we have to develop. It has always been there. It is usually just drowned out by chatter and emotionality. Perhaps you can identify times in your life when it was more frequently noticed.

Practice zooming out, pausing inner chatter, and holding on to clear and quiet perception, awareness of subtlety and intention. If you don't feel anything, that's okay, just practice the two-fold spiritual cycle of integrations: implement targeted awareness on the most interesting thing in each moment, and also relax into trusting expansion.

Let this new seed sprout. Practice holding yourself in highly sensitive states without falling asleep or dropping into internal dialogue. Such a fall is referred to as false identification, or identification with the false self. Instead, stay with the real Self, by any means necessary.

This kind of meditation increases your short-term working memory; it helps you to see the causes of things and notice more thought-associations. To attain measures of success in this pursuit is known as Self-recognition. It is quite a worthy challenge and offers the greatest reward.

The real Self

Some systems of belief posit that there is no real or higher Self, that the nature of human consciousness is of thoughts arising in space without a traceable source. These systems amount to kind of suicide, frankly. Faced with realisation of the error of identifying with the false self — the personality — these systems make an additional jump to abandon the idea that there could even be an integrated whole Self[61].

The Self is real and attainable. It is a "superposition" complete with particles and fields, patterns that permeate the micro and macrocosm, steeped in unconditional love and flourishing evolutionary themes. Look closer, develop your concentration, and you will increasingly know the Self. It is familiar, and in fact it is **of the nature of familiarity**.

It is synesthetic and presents incredible insights much faster than a drawling monologue. If you develop your concentrative awareness, you will know it to be your own true subjectivity. It is an aggregate containing experiences of being a child, recollections of eternality, at times scary feelings of intimacy, swooning rushes of epiphany, and ultimately a sense of knowingness. All these words being inadequate, in Sanskrit it is called *saccidānanda*.

---

[61] Such systems, sometimes called "impersonalist", are very compatible with scientific materialism, and are thus rather popular at the moment.

Put the psychic in front

One may experience clarity of communication from the Self without being tainted by the chitchat of mundane conscious activity. Titan of *yoga* Śrī Aurobindo says to allow the psychic being to come to the front[62], and it requires an active habit of dissociating from chatter so the stream of awareness is uninterrupted. He thus describes the role of a seer, or *ṛṣi*.

Most people can recall experiences of having an epiphany and seeming to "get it" suddenly, having a break-through or realisation. In an instant, we have an experience of greater knowing and a feeling of awe. What was confusing and incomplete suddenly makes sense, and the previous state of uncertainty or frustration is gone. There is a removal of fog, an uplifting awareness of what to do. This can become the daily norm, and continuously attending to the contents of imagination is the key.

People often grown up in an environment where imagination is de-prioritised and a regime of rules-based rote-learning is enforced. When I was a kid, I would occupy myself with my eyes closed laying down exploring visual worlds behind my eyelids. One time, as an adult, I remembered this childhood hobby and thought to do it again. It was troubling to realise I could not! I was out of practice.

Compliance-centric environments result in a stark inability to enable the feeling of excitement. What emerges is a habitual second-guessing of intuition and a disempowering reliance on external sources of motivation and instruction. This situation certainly helps anyone seeking to profit from being the dispensary of things considered necessary for happiness.

---

62 Śrī Aurobindo, *Synthesis of Yoga* (Pondicherry: Sri Aurobindo Ashram Publication 1999)

Self-doubt might look like wisdom sometimes. Many people conflate the two and find themselves erring on the side of inaction, starving their spontaneous, creative, and youthful clarity. This pattern plays out in *yoga* classes as well, where people simply aren't used to the concept of empowered and self-directed action. They seek permission from an external instructor to feel good. Let us learn and move on from this.

In Mysore style classes, students learn to generate their own micro-doses of excitement by persistently moving in a way that is positive and constructive. Each movement is imbued with an earnest sentiment. This is all automatic, you don't have to know about this mechanism or read this book or do any other preparation, all you have to do is show up and practice regularly. Just present yourself to practice under the caring eye of a teacher. Place yourself in a room where you will be adding to a quiet group energy of mutual support.

These practices are radiantly positive and their effects are observed outside of the *yoga* school. We become better versions of ourselves, and others notice too — often before we do.

On any morning of practice, you could have stayed in bed. You could have done a practice at home without any scrutiny. You could have gone to a led class where the task of motivation is outsourced to an instructor and self-intimacy is rewduced. **But you chose this.**

Every time you attend a Mysore style class, your sense of autonomy and bearing is bolstered. You have the dawning realisation that you are in control of your mind, energy levels, emotions, responses and actions. Where you may have once felt like a victim of existence with feelings of despair and resentment, you now automatically select positive postures in your life.

You re-identify yourself as the author of every moment and are entirely capable of creating positive effects. You are empowered and it keeps getting easier and more automatic over time.

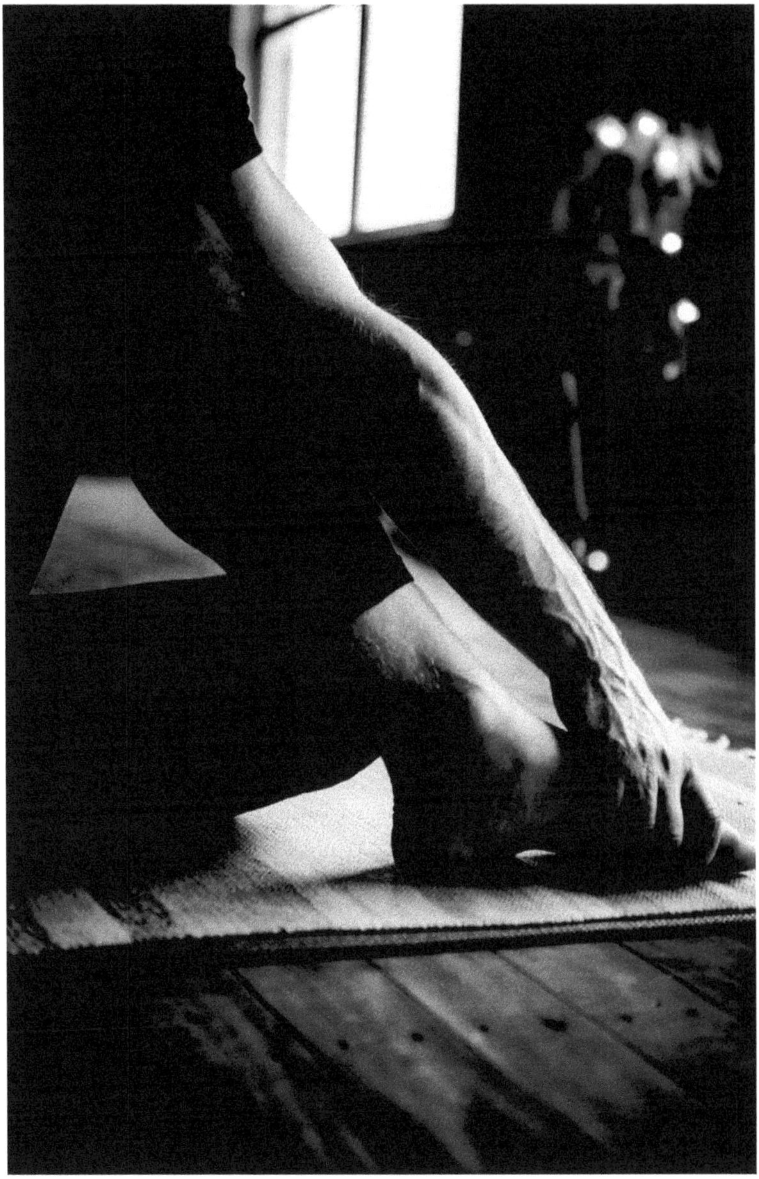

Photo credit: Kate Binnie

6

ADVANCED YOGA

In Ashtanga Vinyasa Yoga, we learn to establish strong roots with the primary series, and then stretch our branches out and grow tall as can be with the intermediate series.

Sensitivity is cultivated and we sincerely embrace all that we encounter with the assumption that it serves us positively, even when not immediately apparent. All the while there is a song in the heart and an irresistible playfulness in daily life.

The third series contains, predictably, more challenging forward bends and back bends. In addition, there is a large focus on arm balances and handstands. It is called in Sanskrit *sthira bhāga*, meaning "stable or resolute happiness". When the trunk is straight and firm, the leaves and flowers can writhe and twinkle through the seasons.

To be a pillar of society

The third series has been declared to be for the purpose of demonstration, and this is a gladdening statement that helps reduce the focus on needing to accomplish such extreme poses. There is a more nuanced truth to the statement as well:

The advanced series is for demonstration of the spiritual process.

During the practice of *yoga* thus far, the understanding ought to have unfolded that acts in service of others are also acts of service to Self, since those others are located within the Self. The habit of unbounded service has thus naturally developed, and we desire to act as a conscious creator. Now we stand tall, resolute in the centre, while adaptable and spontaneous in the periphery.

Identify with *śiva* at the top of the mountain, possessing ultimate awareness and ultimate will that dwarfs the unruly tendencies of the surface mind. You can live there. When you live there, you don't so much feel "different" — **you feel more like you**. All of your sojourns and lives-within-lives are here and now, present and available. You **are now** five years old, and 12 years, and 18, and 80. All of your perspectives are here.

To become *śiva* and see with completeness and balance, you must have discovered and addressed the neglected parts within you, any disturbances that cause you to become disharmonious. The method can be as simple and physical as learning to breathe with smooth and even character while standing on one leg, or to balance on your hands upside down with your eyes closed. This has staggering potency and it ultimately must be directly experienced rather than discussed.

Make truth the native state of the mind. Set up the mind so that nothing but truth can exist within it. Persistently set a clear intention for self-honesty and then travel along the path, discovering all of your polarities so they can be neutralised and balanced by viewing their opposite.

Here is the two-phase spiritual cycle we have been exploring: aim for the top of the mountain, or a place that seems virtuous and adventurous, and then invest effort in persistently moving in this direction, surrendering to the practice of resolving polarities as they arise.

Reinvention and transformation

Through the process of *yoga*, primal hesitancy transforms. Fear of falling seems to be removed. It must be experienced to be understood. At a very fundamental level, you know that your body will take care of itself in situations of mortal peril. This is the posture called *samasthiti*.

In order to become a healer, you must be well along the path of resolving, in yourself, the biases of life up to this point. You must know what you actually are — an energetic signature in consciousness that creates apparitions of personality. You must be symmetrical, axial, capable of bending in any direction. You must move in harmony with the wave-motion that underpins all, while simultaneously being poised in the centre.

What an incredible time to be alive, to be so free and able to reinvent ourselves frequently. Revere the reformers from long ago and those in the current age. Musical artists like David Bowie and Mike Patton are pioneers here, wilfully discarding the past and reinventing for the sake of something new and fertile.

We are compelled to keep reinventing ourselves. We are urged to embrace the feeling of being unbounded and unsecured, with a trust in the natural order, the evolutionary process, and that positivity attracts positivity. To be bold and beyond convention. To make the decision that we can have it all, and that our active imagination is the key motive force.

Faith, belief, assumption — these are synonyms. Faith is the default operating system of the human being. Colossal decisions are made based on inference. We rely on information from people who, empirically, we cannot prove exist. We take it for granted that they exist. We refer to memory and senses that are apparently subject to bias and fabrication. When you get out of bed in the morning, you immediately employ faith that things will be a certain way, that the floor will be there, and that it is now the day after yesterday. Faith underpins all of our actions. An unflinching trust in our own assumptions. Nothing is solid.

To be unaware that you are pretending is blindness.

To be aware is to empower yourself to create your desired viewpoint.

You may feel like it is difficult to create and maintain your desired viewpoint, as though it takes effort and is thus tiring and fraught. But this too is a voluntary belief. We are already being faithful, all the time, to a certain viewpoint. Faith is not something to develop, it is the way we always operate. We load assumptions about reality and execute them faithfully, often never interrogating them once they are set up.

We have been conditioned to believe that we are nothing but a curious emergent property of biological structures. We have been trained to think of ourselves as intelligent flesh robots, subject to the whims of circumstance. Dominated by the material world, we are tasked with ensuring the best material circumstances for ourselves in the face of billions of other people also trying to attain that for themselves.

The materialist assumption is that humans are creatures with very limited control over their world and over their inner lives, unable to trust the accuracy of their minds and senses, locked within an external world that constantly infringes upon them. This creates widespread, if quiet, fear and angst. It is a selected world view, as we have discussed, and it forces people to become bellicose or submissive.

Teaching people this powerlessness from infancy creates a situation where they must seek to either enhance their power and dominate, or to protect their paltry interests by surrendering their will to a force that can dominate on their behalf. Over time, a Stockholm Syndrome appears where people begin to defend their captor. The doctrine of scarcity is a dogma peddled by materialist culture that inculcates children with the perspective that reality is limited to what is perceptible with the senses and analysable with the intellect. Other views are cast aside as primitive or delusional.

Even when mind is found to affect matter, it is labelled "placebo" and summarily pushed aside. When people wish to continue exploring beyond, they are met with sneers or ostracised. The notion that matter is directly affected by, or emerges from, consciousness is an afront to the surface mind. Similarly, ideas around co-location of physical forms, entanglement of particles, and other adventures of jumping around time-space with no regard for linearity, are a threat that must (at least initially) be shut down, ridiculed, and de-funded in academia. Nonetheless, while these limitations act as a drag on evolution, the laudable adherence to pure logic by the modern sciences means that eventually, inch-by-inch, reality beyond the parameters of three-dimensional space and mono-directional time must be faced.

The begrudging loosening of assumptions is the same behaviour that we have seen in organised religion. When such an institution is confronted with undeniable evidence, they make bare-minimum shifts in the direction of truth. When it comes to the crunch of personal illness, for example, priests will tend to take advantage of medical science, just as they claim atheists turn to a sky-god when facing death in a foxhole.

Our corporate-science culture is compelled to use the equations of quantum mechanics to develop new technologies, even though the way it works is not completely understood. The pursuit of this understanding attracts only a guarded and token support in universities.

We have recreated a class of mystics who explore the scary things on our behalf while we go about our mundane lives. It used to be priests and shamans, now it's theoretical physicists. We ask them to open the door and experience the pregnant void of paradoxes on our behalf, and they return to us with fables and illustrations of their journeys.

Something to dazzle us in our free time.

It is the spirit of the matter.

Act as though

The way to counter a rigid belief that you are a player within an "outside world" is to think and act in the opposite manner, starting with *āsana*. Instead of viewing your body as something that you are subject to, something that you are encumbered by, view it as something that you alone created and that you are recreating in every moment.

When you attempt to perform a handstand, for example, and happen to notice that you cannot do a handstand, interrupt any automatic beliefs and thoughts that follow the failed attempt. Interrupt any tendency to collect evidence to reinforce the assumption that you cannot do handstands. Instead, insert the opposite belief — that you **are able** to do handstands, that the capacity is **temporarily forgotten**, and that you simply are allowing this skill to be remembered by your playful physical creation called "the body".

Then, in an act of persistent positivity, repeatedly practice handstands with the expectation that fully remembering the skill is inevitable. The temporary omission of handstanding ability in your life will pass.

Maintain the decision that **you can** do a handstand and that you are particularly well-suited to doing handstands. Gradually notice evidence to support this. Along the way you will uncover things that need to be addressed, such as strength, or flexibility, or patience and determination.

Actively notice every time you seem to be more capable. Look for positive evidence. There are many pieces of proof that only you can access. We have trained ourselves to discard subjective data, calling it cognitive bias. But **everything** is cognitive bias!

You tend to notice evidence that supports your beliefs. Use this as a tool for your advantage. You are always reinforcing your worldview, so select it consciously. Take the time to notice that you are improving each day, and use this evidence to become emboldened. Restate your decision over and over. Understand through your own direct experience that you are creating your own bodily reality.

The intellect that previously gave you thoughts of not being strong enough or not having the right body type for this-or-that can be proven wrong through direct experience. The intellect is frequently wrong, actually. When it is placed in charge of the entire being, it is forced to try and predict the future. It becomes hyper-vigilant and susceptible to guilt and fear. But you need not believe negative suggestions when they arise, and it's wise to cultivate awareness of when they subtly slide in, uninvited.

This process of creating beliefs (and therefore reality) becomes increasingly fun. You move to the mountaintop more frequently by dissolving polarities, and you tend to stay there more often. Let the intellect narrate what **has happened** while you set up what **will happen** with your higher functions — your intention and imagination.

The word *bhāvana* indicates the induction of a state or a thing through progressive, repetitive, cultivating actions. This is a purpose of many ritualistic activities seen in *yoga*. It can even manifest as becoming "worked up" in a whirl of enthusiasm. This consistent aspiration is our fuel and we contain an unlimited supply, although an exclusively material mindset cannot help but be encumbered by ideas of lack and scarcity.

Some activities for whipping up enthusiasm might be viewed as strange — singing and chanting on the street for example — but it takes a certain amount of daring to shed all that self-doubt and conservatism.

The 18th century text Ātma Vidyā Vilāsa explains the symptoms of residing in high level awareness (called "nondualism" or *advaita*) while operating in the world of separateness (called "dualism" or *dvaita*). It notes that the great aspirants who know the truth (that all apparently external forms actually exist within your universally large body) wander about like a fool, unaware of any difference between creatures, seeing only one.

Cynicism is common when the intellect is appointed as leader of the entity. Legendary punk and poet, Henry Rollins, speaks about the build-up of cynicism he experienced living in America and knowing so many people who died from murder, suicide, misadventure and overdose:

> *"I came to realise that cynicism is intellectual cowardice. It's not taking the time to deal with what is. It was so much fun being cynical but I can't do it anymore. I don't want to turn into some floating Buddha, that's not me either but I think one must strive to bear the heavy lift of objectivity. It's hard work not being cynical. You have to listen to both sides of every argument. It sucks sometimes but that's what it takes."*

It can be disheartening to see religious folk and cults who appear intoxicated by their own wishful thinking. In society we also see raving lunatics, new-age crystal coddlers, drug-addled hippies, and the corporate personal-development charlatans selling the ability to sell.

Seeing all of this, it would be easy to write off the notion of sculpting circumstances in your life through excursions in the imagination. But ironically, writing off the notion of sculpting life through your beliefs is a demonstration of that same behaviour.

To write it off would be to clamp down and appoint the basic, fearful, sceptical, superstitious, tribal mind as the supreme arbiter of truth. It would be a decision to relegate joyous creativity to youth, artists, and crazy people. So often people decide to embrace creativity only when it is materially justified, once all of the "more important" jobs have been done.

But we need to be impassioned in increasing measure — we want to bounce out of bed in the morning. We want to employ the basic brain for tasks at which it excels — those of a procedural nature. This frees us up to work predominantly in the imagination. The neurotic babbling of the surface mind has managed to populate our attention so much that it's easy to forget that anything else exists in consciousness.

> *"I spent most of my life being angry and frustrated and cynical and pessimistic because my heart was constantly broken by what I saw in the world. Gradually this turned to apathy and nihilism in order to protect myself. Eventually I realised that the world needs my intensity, be it in the form of fury or pain or deep empathy — it is the apathy that deadens us and allows us to become automatons as we age. Seeing only the brutality of the world is tiring"*
> – *Mysore student.*

Consider emotions like sincerity, confidence, and ardour. This is what we are in essence, that is what we are made of. Pure unbridled consciousness is exemplified by the word "yes". It is unlimited permissiveness, willingness, adventure. It is where we go to have peak experiences.

It gets easier and easier to re-integrate and re-member our native attitude. The inner truth of our being is a fountain of wildly positive feelings. If you want to have access to all of your mind and all of your body you will need to become comfortable with feeling good **at all times**, even when society says you should "look busy".

You are allowed to select and identify with infinite love every moment, without conditions. It is your birthright to unfold like this. In every moment you are using your will to express a chosen set of assumptions. It may be unconscious and automatic, nonetheless you are doing it. In *yoga* we employ physical techniques to train the habit of selecting our state.

Body language matters a great deal — when we practice bold physical postures, we repeatedly induce a non-verbal understanding of our power to choose the positive view and the integrative action in every situation.

To balance on our hands is a dramatic gesture of this poised intention. To reflexively **burst into laughter** while doing something scary is to reinforce our true nature as playful in the extreme.

This is the spirit of spontaneity needed to live a healthy life of creative joy. It is the natural result of the spiritual process: the combination of *abhyāsa* (concentrative practice) and *vairāgya* (relaxed dis-identification).

Take rest

I have the privilege of witnessing people come to *yoga* for the first time. It is commonly observed that new people have difficulty laying still. Often there is noticeable twitching and fidgeting during a simple five-minute rest at the end of practice. This is emblematic of a society that induces a mild version of post-traumatic stress disorder (PTSD) in response to living the prescribed life.

Thankfully, we just as often see a removal of this tension over a modest period of time practicing *yoga*. People are able to relax more deeply, and they reclaim the ability to have a simple rest during the day.

It is possible to accrue a militant attitude when we uncritically accept the idea that reality originates from a mythical outside place and that we are helpless to resist its incursions upon us. The felt need to survive can elicit behaviours such as allowing ourselves or others to be hurt — glossing over pain in the body or allowing poor people to starve on the streets of big cities — there's no time to complain, no time for self-care.

In order to balance this and replace habits of denial, practices of *yoga* involving intense watching are used. Attention is placed on the Self, which is **one whole thing** that contains the individual personality and the projected external world. Even your physical body is inside you. True strength and eternal safety are found in this clear vision.

You are always dreaming. Dreams are always occurring. Imagination is the canvas upon which all of reality exists. All experiences — mundane sense perceptions, eyes-open dreams, and eyes-closed dreams — all of these appear on the same field of imagination, and it is a playground containing vast information.

You probably have a strong bias towards thinking in words and sentences. It can be overcome, and this is the skill developed in meditation. Allow inner chatter to subside so that the images become obvious. Watch those forms dance without slipping into commentary. During *āsana* practice do less talking in your head and pay more attention to the dream state. Notice that dreams occur when you are awake. Take control of your consciousness and make it your craft.

Rather incredible things happen over the years, as you do this. Parts of yourself become noticed and integrated, parts that were separated, disowned, forgotten. Clairvoyant people often observe that a child version of a person hangs around the adult, and they gradually merge as the spiritual journey progresses.

In the rest of this chapter, we will explore more techniques from the traditions of *yoga* that launch us into subtle planes, using the energising stability of *āsana* as a foundation. But keep in mind that many profound experiences require nothing more than a simple 15-minute lay down called *śavāsana* — a great opportunity to freely explore consciousness.

Explore the interstices

Positions of deep relaxation while awake can help us explore states of absorption, like the one called *nāda anusandhāna* in Yoga Tārāvalī.

There are many such techniques in the canon of *yoga*. The ancient text Tripurā Rahasya gives examples where states of absorption are found in ordinary life: when a person is embraced for the first time by their new and beloved wife, or when they suddenly acquire something for which they have long hankered, or when they are feeling happily carefree and suddenly come across a life-threatening danger like a tiger, or when they hear that their son has unexpectedly died.

All of these moments describe the sudden removal of distinction between inner consciousness and the projected outside world consisting of time and space. Crucially, these are also waking experiences, intense enough to prevent the person being overcome by sleep (the tendency to accidentally fall asleep is well known).

Another technique is listed in Tripurā Rahasya for entering the state of absorption that does not require such intense worldly situations. It is explained that *samādhi* can be found in the intervals between the ordinary states of human consciousness. That is, there is a transition point between waking and sleeping, and with practice it can be expanded to last a very long time. This particular practice is also known as *yoga nidrā*.

Let us uncover the Yoga Tārāvalī on the ensuing right-hand pages of this chapter. You may read the text by itself by flicking through each verse, or you may read it in amongst the rest of chapter six. Note that I have added additional explanatory comments in square brackets [ ].

Yoga Tārāvalī – योगतारावली

śloka 1

वन्दे गुरूणां चरणारविन्दे संदर्शितस्वात्मसुखावबोधे।
जनस्य ये जाङ्गलिकायमाने संसार हालाहल मोहशान्त्यऐ॥

vande gurūṇāṃ caraṇāravinde saṁdarśitasvātmasukhāvabodhe ।
janasya ye jāṅgalikāyamāne saṃsāra hālāhala mohaśāntyai ॥

I revere this, the vision of the true Self, which is revealed at the feet of the *guru*-s. This vision causes joyful condition and all the good circumstances. It is the snake-charmer that neutralises the deadly poison of false-identity, the delusion of *saṃsāra*, for the peace of humanity.

śloka 2

सदाशिवोक्तानि सपादलक्ष लयावधानानि वसन्ति लोके।
नादानुसंधानसमाधिमेकं मन्यामहे मान्यतमं लयानाम्॥

sadāśivoktāni sapādalakṣa layāvadhānāni vasanti loke ।
nādānusaṁdhāna samādhimekaṃ manyāmahe mānyatamaṃ layānām ॥

The perpetually existent highest Self of all, called *śiva*, promulgates for us in the material world, innumerable types of absorptive focus [directing us to the universal origin of time and form]. The particular kind involving intense investigation on the inner sound, *nāda*, we declare best of all.

Active sleep

In the modern marketplace, *yoga nidrā* it has come to refer to a very specific stage-by-stage relaxation of the body in order to find this threshold between waking and sleeping. Historically, the term is a little broader and can overlap with the word *samādhi.* It translates as "un-inert sleep" — a very active waking state with the eyes closed.

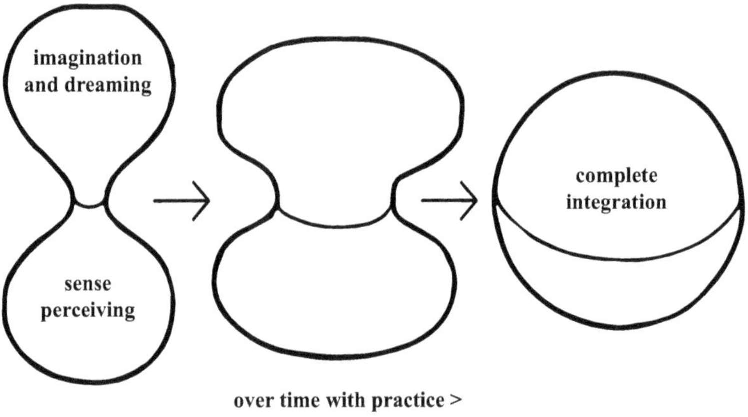

Diagram: Blending the sense perceptible and the imagination together over time.

The more you do *yoga nidrā* and the other techniques we are exploring, the easier it gets. You open the aperture, gently float up to the ceiling, and pop your head through the manhole.

In the process, you are exercise devotion by over-riding the tendency to sleep. You are maintaining your position at the lotus feet of the goddess. The vitalising nectar of dreams drips into your waking consciousness.

A very effective method to get a handle on this is to wake from your nightly sleep and hover in the half-awake twilight. It can be advantageous to set your alarm for an hour earlier than you normally wake, so that you may lay longer in the semi-dreaming state.

With practice you can leave the door to the dreaming state open for hours.

śloka 3

सरेचपूरऐरनलिस्य कुम्भऐःसर्वासु नाडीषु वशिोधतिास।
अनाहताख्यो बहुभःिप्रकारऐरन्तःप्रवर्तेत सदा ननिादः॥

sa recapūrairanilasya kumbhaiḥ sarvāsu nāḍīṣu viśodhitāsu ।
anāhatākhyo bahubhiḥ prakārairantaḥ pravarteta sadā ninādaḥ ॥

As one cleanses all the channels of the body, called *nadi*-s, by inhalation, exhalation, and breath retention, then the many kinds of unstruck sounds, [audible sounds without physical cause], *anāhata*, increase continuously.

śloka 4

नादानुसंधान नमोऽस्तु तुभ्यं त्वां साधनं तत्त्वपदस्य जाने।
भवत्प्रसादात्पवनेन साकं वलीयते वष्णिुपदे मनो मे॥

nādānusaṁdhāna namo'stu tubhyaṃ tvāṃ sādhanaṃ tattvapadasya jāne ।
bhavatprasādātpavanena sākaṃ vilīyate viṣṇupade mano me ॥

Oh *nāda*, how glorious is your examination! Truly, we should petition you [to allow sounds above and below the perceptible spectrum of the physical sense organs to infringe upon our waking consciousness]. Mastering you delivers access to the subtle causes while remaining in this material life. By grace, and by bringing in the [unsettled oscillations of] energy, little-by-little we adhere to the co-locative feet of *viṣṇu*, [which is the bridge to the non-physical, that place beyond places, the reservoir of knowledge-bliss and natural free will].

A great deal happens in dream consciousness, but it occurs so quickly it tends to be missed. Such a large portion of life does not have to be lost in a haze. We can learn to maintain focus on the both eyes-open and eyes-closed worlds at once.

The challenge of staying awake on the edge of dreaminess is the reason it's usually advised to sit upright while meditating. The goal is to go into that non-verbal imagination space quickly, to be able to dive in at will while you are awake.

Practicing *yoga āsana* in a Mysore style setting also helps. When you practice in a quietly introverted yet physically active manner immediately after waking — doing the same postures every day, without someone loudly instructing you every step of the way — you can close your eyes and dream while moving and breathing through the poses.

You can pay attention to what is always there but usually missed in sleep.

Mystical sound and vision

In these practices of dwelling at the borderline, we develop a peculiar kind of concentration. Note that the word "concentrate" is usually treated as a verb — a task to be done. But it can be used as a noun — as in a liquid concentrate, a pool of substance from which thoughts and actions arise.

The term *dhyāna* means the uninterrupted flow of remembrance or information, it is the accumulation of concentration from an object. As one stops identifying with thoughts and actions, remaining focused on the subtle source, the concentrate increases. The experience is of a welling up, a sense of being so established in that place that you no longer want to indulge in lower-level distraction.

The material world will always remain easily accessible, so allow yourself to be distracted by higher-level workings instead for a change. This is the meaning of *nāda anusandhāna*.

Śloka 5

जालन्धरोड्याणनमूलबन्धाञ्जल्पन्ति कण्ठोदरपायुमूलात।
बन्धत्रयेऽस्मिन्परिचीयमाने बन्धःकुतो दारुणकालपाशात॥

jālandharoḍyāṇamūlabandhāñjalpanti kaṇṭhodarapāyumūlāt ।
bandhatraye'sminparicīyamāne bandhaḥ kuto dāruṇakālapāśāt ॥

The *bandha*-s are known by their physical locations of the throat, abdomen, and pelvic floor, [and we culture the material body using these instruments, exercising the physical to vivify the spiritual]. When these psycho-physical bridging mechanisms are consistently engaged, [the artifice of an exclusively material existence becomes untenable, and] no longer can the cruel snare of [incessantly sequential] space-time catch us!

Śloka 6

ओड्याणजालन्धरमूलबन्धएैरुन्नद्रितायामुरगाङ्गनायाम।
प्रत्यङ्मुखत्वात्प्रवशिन्सुषुम्नां गमागमऔ मुञ्चतगिन्धवाहः॥

oḍyāṇajālandharamūlabandhairunnidritāyāmuragāṅganāyām ।
pratyaṅgamukhatvātpraviśansuṣumnāṃ gamāgamau muñcati gandhavāhaḥ ॥

When the earthen base is firmly sealed, the water-spout is consciously contained, and the pumping mechanism is elastic and strong, the beautiful serpentine form may arise from the dormant state [of obliviousness to the spirit, with incongruent patterns of the superficial mind predominating, along with entropy and the condition of birth and death]. From her downcast state, *kuṇḍalinī* enters the central channel of *suṣumṇa*, and the effects of [those scattered] comings and goings are left behind.

Non-physical sounds and visual content blend into barely describable nebulae within consciousness. Such ideations are the doorway to higher forms, so we meditate upon them. Spheres of consciousness are available to us that seem at times alien to the fixed physical personality with which we are accustomed.

The tiring compulsion to talk and fuss is replaced by important revelations and spiritual experience. It must be experienced to be understood. It is to be seated in awareness of the over-arching order of formerly contradictory things, resulting in a sense of peace and power.

In this way, *yoga* is the skill of seeing and hearing that which is always present. You are already totally immersed in the famous bliss of *nirvana*, and now is a good time to open to it and to be aware of what obscures your enjoyment of it. A complete blending of the worlds is sought — both the ordinary and seemingly external physical world, as well as the spiritual world of images and dream content.

In neuroscience, physics, and cosmology there are interesting and provocative theories which posit the nature of reality to be purely mathematical, or that we are living in a simulation, or that all human experience is a hallucination (ie. the perception of something not present). This easily turns into a debate about definitions and assumptions.

Yoga agrees with the value of this line of questioning. In my experience, this is the most entertaining and energising topic that young and curious minds alike gravitate to. Unfortunately, it is often replaced by more mundane, "productive", activity as adulthood and materiality takes hold. Not only does *yoga* endorse the excavation of such topics, it also takes the endeavour to its logical end by advocating simultaneous awareness of all universes, planes, fields, functions, and particles.

śloka 7

उत्थापिताधारहुताशनोल्कऐराकुञ्चनऐःशश्वदपानवायोः।
सन्तापिताच्चन्द्रमसःपतन्ती पीयूषधारां पबितीह धन्यः ॥

utthāpitādhārahutāśanolkairākuñcanaiḥ śaśvadapānavāyoḥ I
saṁtāpitāccandramasaḥ patantī pīyūṣadhārāṃ pibatīha dhanyaḥ II

By means of the powerfully arousing action of fire, caused by contortion of the physical body, the downward facing energy is compressed and rotates to rise upwards. The ambrosial moon at the head [the reservoir of piety and humaniform potential, which is joined to the glands of the skull, and can be excited with the tongue] becomes over-heated, and an overflow of nectar thus streams, to be drunk, bestowing fortune.

śloka 8

बन्धत्रयाभ्यासवपिाकजातां ववर्जितां रेचकपूरकाभ्याम।
वशिोषयन्तीं वषियप्रवाहं वद्यिां भजे केवलकुम्भरूपाम ॥

bandhatrayābhyāsavipākajātāṃ vivarjitāṃ recakapūrakābhyām I
viśoṣayantīṃ viṣayapravāhaṃ vidyāṃ bhaje kevalakumbharūpām II

With the ripening practice of the three-fold *bandha*, devoid of inhale and exhale, comes the burning up of the flow of mental constructs [as disharmony loses its support]. I thus honour the appearance [marked by revelatory flashes] of spontaneous suspension that is *kevala kumbhaka*.

At the beginning, it is enough to just discover that there is such an elaborate spiritual world and to take more serious looks. Next comes the ability to go there quickly and to derive tangible benefit from it. Eventually an admixture appears and both occupy the same space, removing the need to switch between them. Such spontaneous fusion, this breathtaking suspension, is called *kevala kumbhaka.*

Techniques relating to non-physical sound and vision are a terrific way to explore blending. They enable us to align the levels of physical apparatus, to shorten the path between external and internal, to widen the conduit, so that sensing is more directly performed by the mind itself. The intermediaries we call sense organs are "purified" or "opened" to the extent that they present no further obstacle, friction, time lag, or filter.

Those physical senses are middle men, reaching from the "outer" objects to one single meeting place in the brain. This meeting place is the master sense or the root sense, called *manas.* This is where mental perception occurs, and when the physical senses are purified and effectively made redundant, *manas* becomes the sole sense organ.

The techniques we are describing share a common characteristic where the sense faculty receives vastly more energy and attention than usual, an overflow of sorts. Focus expands from the mundane object being perceived to the organ involved in sensing. Then, on to the root sensory function of the brain, and to the act of perception itself. It's a little like repeating a word over and over until the label loses all meaning. There is a sustained effort to disorient normal functioning until a different mode is established. The mind is fixed on an object until names and labels dissolve, leaving only true context and accurate knowledge.

With diligent practice, a series of break-throughs are made where the mind moves through progressively more subtle states of perception. It follows the same two-stage cyclical process of piercing super-concentration, followed by rushes of observant expansion.

śloka 9

अनाहते चेतसि सावधानैरभ्यासशूरैरनुभूयमाना ।
संस्तम्भित श्वासमनःप्रचारा सा जृम्भते केवलकुम्भकश्रीः ॥

anāhate cetasi sāvadhānairabhyāsaśūrairanubhūyamānā ।
saṃstambhita śvāsamanaḥ pracārā sā jṛmbhate kevalakumbhakaśrīḥ ॥

It is by persistent attention on the non-physical sounds that conscientious students experience such paralysis of breath and mind. One then receives the lightning radiance of *kevala kumbhaka,* [apprehended in body and senses, bestowing greater expression of state-change].

śloka 10

सहस्रशःसन्तु हठेषु कुम्भाःसम्भाव्यते केवलकुम्भ एव ।
कुम्भोत्तमे यत्र तु रेचपूरौ प्राणस्य न प्राकृतवैकृताख्यौ ॥

sahasraśaḥ santu haṭheṣu kumbhāḥ sambhāvyate kevalakumbha eva ।
kumbhottame yatra tu recapūrau prāṇasya na prākṛtavaikṛtākhyau ॥

Of all the thousands of *kumbhaka* in *haṭha yoga*, this one stands alone. There, in the loftiest of suspensions, the comings and goings of *prāṇa* cannot be called intentional nor distracted, not interesting nor boring, not normal nor abnormal. [All particles of *prakṛti* are seen in their neutrality, resting in their transitory state, waiting for you to assign meaning].

Over and over, we practice bubbling up to successive new planes. Each plane contains vastly more content than the preceding one, the surface mind becomes less involved, and we move into states that feel like dreaming with rich conscious content. The mundane experience is relegated so profoundly that it can knock us into an actual physical sleep, which ought to be avoided, lest we lose the practice.

Trāṭaka is a tool that can reveal to us just how vivid and rapturous meditation can be — a far cry from sitting still and trying to become blank. Instead, revelations of heretofore hidden dimensions are visible.

To practice *trāṭaka*, place your attention on some physical object and do not blink. Allow your mind to be completely focused on the object. Notice any inner dialogue and allow it to subside. Initially, this is a fairly physical exercise of controlling the eyeballs and coping with the discomfort of not blinking. You are awake and sitting with your eyes open, so you will not fall asleep.

As the mind settles, the space between your eyeballs and the object becomes more interesting. You will see your imagination with your eyes open. Cascades of effects are realised, and once found they can be accessed again rather easily without the former strain.

Look inside your skull

In Tripurā Rahasya, the author describes stretching the vision so as to notice the spaces in between the perceiver and the apparent object.

You can try it: with a concentrated mind, see some object in the distance, and understand that it is within your very own consciousness that extends far beyond the human form. Notice how much space you actually occupy. All things are within you. This is to open the borders and allow the master sense to directly perceive with less translation from the sense organs.

śloka 11

त्रकिूटनाम्नि स्तिमितिऽन्तरङ्गे खे स्तंभति केवलकुम्भकेन ।
प्राणानलिो भानुशशाङ्कनाड्यौ वहिाय सद्यो वलियं प्रयातिा॥

trikūṭanāmni stimite'ntaraṅge khe staṁbhite kevalakumbhakena I
prāṇānilo bhānuśaśāṅkanāḍyau vihāya sadyo vilayaṃ prayāti II

The introverted and motionless space called *trikūṭa* [the high point on the mountain where the rivers originate at three mouths: the solar, lunar, and the thin central channel], is accessed during this paralysis of oscillation. Even the very subtlest wavering tendencies, wisps of scattered *prāṇa*, move beyond the scope of polarised solar and lunar urges, and are immediately rejoined in the central command.

śloka 12

प्रत्याहृ्तः केवलकुम्भकेन प्रबुद्ध कुण्डल्युपभुक्तशेषः ।
प्राणःप्रतीचीनपथेन मन्दं वलीियते वष्णिुपदान्तराळे ॥

pratyāhṛtaḥ kevalakumbhakena prabuddha kuṇḍalyupabhuktaśeṣaḥ I
prāṇaḥ pratīcīnapathena mandaṃ vilīyate viṣṇupadāntarāḷe II

Held in the home of the heart, the highest junction, by means of *kevala kumbhaka*, nascent *kuṇḍalinī* awakens and swallows up residual *prāṇa*, [moving it up to integration, letting go of disharmony, argumentation, and conditioning], inducing it as a vortex via *suṣumṇa* into *viṣṇu*, [the unconditioned infinite where reconciliation occurs with ease].

In Ashtanga Vinyasa Yoga a mild version of visual concentration is performed. Similar to *trāṭaka*, it is called *dṛṣṭi* and it involves controlling the movement of the eyeballs for five breaths at a time. Each pose has a prescribed focal point, usually it's the tip of the nose, the thumb, the sky, navel etc. During *āsana* you practice staring at one thing only. On a surface level, this *dṛṣṭi* helps you rein in the wandering mind by having a fixed gaze. But *dṛṣṭi* is really a warm-up for seated *trāṭaka* practice that spans several minutes. With this training regimen you will be more readily able to tap directly into previously hidden aspects of consciousness — all of this occurring during a quiet, Mysore style practice.

A very special technique, *śāmbhavī mudrā*, goes further by peering **into** the third eye while the eyelids are open. That is, one focuses the visual sense on an area in the centre of the skull. In a way, it is a visual form of interoception. This time, the focal point is between the eyeballs and back into the skull — the region of the third ventricle of the brain known as the ambrosial moon. Point the gaze inside the brain while the eyelids are open to see subtle consciousness overlaid upon the sense perceptions.

When *śāmbhavī* is implemented, the radiance of the underlying substrate, *brahman*, is unveiled. It filters into waking consciousness as a white and black glow, like lightning or a strobe light[63]. I used to read descriptions like those in the Yoga Tārāvalī and other texts and think "how lovely is the poetry", then I had the direct experience and understood what is meant. To explain any further effects at this point would be to jump the gun and possibly place suggestions in the path of your own native experience. It is best that you do the practice earnestly and innocently.

---

[63] This technique liberates one from residing exclusively in the material world. In fact, the higher Self is said to be possessed of infinite and recursive illumination, and can thus maintain the principal physical body even while a *yogi* leaves it to go on journeys (Bṛhadāraṇyaka Upanishad 4:3:12)

śloka 13

नरिङ्कुशानां श्वसनोद्गमानां नरिोधन्ऐःकेवलकुम्भकाख्य्ऐः ।
उदेतसिर्वेन्द्रयिवृत्तशिून्यो मरुल्लयःकोऽपमिहामतीनाम ॥

niraṅkuśānāṃ śvasanodgamānāṃ nirodhanaiḥ kevalakumbhakākhyaiḥ I
udeti sarvendriyavṛttiśūnyo marullayaḥ ko 'pi mahāmatīnām II

As even incoming tumult is restrained by the gift of *kevala kumbhaka*, there occurs for the great-minded ones [who seek the swift liberation of knowledge and clarity] a drying-up of all scattered sensations to their ultimate nullification [as the irrecoverable deluge transforms divisiveness into harmonious super-imposition, revealing the expansive shining of diluvian conflagration, the brilliant and transcendent peerless one, resplendent like the effulgence of ten million suns].

śloka 14

न दृष्टलिक्ष्याणनि चत्तिबन्धो न देशकाल्औ न च वायुरोधः ।
न धारणाध्यानपरश्रिमो वा समेधमाने सतरािजयोगे ॥

na dṛṣṭilakṣyāṇi na cittabandho na deśakālau na ca vāyurodhaḥ I
na dhāraṇādhyānapariśramo vā samedhamāne sati rājayoge II

For those thriving and succeeding in this *raja yoga*, there is no longer any visual focus, no mental target, no sense of time or place, no conscious restraining of breath, nor labour of concentration. [The inertia of exclusively physical existence lessens as the peace beneath is seen].

The fourth state

The Upanishads outline three ordinary states of mind: being awake with sense perception (*viṣaya*), observing imagination and dreams (*taijasa*), and deep dreamless sleep (*prajñā*). There is also a fourth state, a super-state, one that is always activated and never falls asleep (*turīya*). It is by means of super-visual *śāmbhavī mudrā* of Maṇḍala Brahman Upanishad and the super-auditory *nāda anusandhāna* of Yoga Tārāvalī that we nimbly traverse the three ordinary states with a view to reaching the fourth.

Since all that you experience occurs on the same conscious field, why not have clear vision of your imagination and the sense perceptions at the same time, without switching between them? Why, also, don't we heed the advice of the ancient scientists and notice that there is an over-arching wakefulness that has always been online — when you were a baby, and when you were elderly, and at all the other moments.

All kinds of samādhi are possible

The highest state, the abode of *śiva*, which goes by many names including *samādhi*, is described in so many ways and yet no description can be adequate. Nonetheless, thousands have attempted to describe it, sometimes as a way of reminding themselves, and sometimes to encourage others to pursue the same state.

In his work titled Samadhi: The Great Freedom, Gregor Maehle explains eight **objective** *samādhi*-s and the ultimate **objectless** *samādhi*, the super-cognitive *samādhi*. He essentially describes a training protocol, a gradation of concentrative targets, and the techniques and underpinning concepts needed to establish an intellectual footing. Having refined the physical mind and body through *āsana* and *prāṇāyāma* to the extent that it can be reliably pressed into a higher service, we give it certain tasks. Foci of increasingly subtle kinds are chosen, and practices of latching onto them in an unbroken state of information transfer are explored.

śloka 15

अशेषदृ्श्योज्झितदृङ्मयानाम अवस्थितानामहि राजयोगे ।
न जागरो नापि सुषुप्तभिावो न जीवतिं नो मरणं वचित्रिम ॥

aśeṣadṛśyojjhitadṛṅmayānām avasthitānāmiha rājayoge ।
na jāgaro nāpi suṣuptibhāvo na jīvitaṃ no maraṇaṃ vicitram ॥

Those established in this *raja yoga*, having moved entirely beyond the seen and taking the pure form of the seer are liberated. For them there is no experience of waking or sleeping, indeed there is not even living or dying — how interesting! [They become flux, of the nature of the field. The separative personality scrambles to latch, but cannot, so is eventually content to trust. Trembling intimacy is the wondrous consequence].

śloka 16

अहंममत्वाद्व्यपहाय सर्व श्रीराजयोगे स्थरिमानसानाम ।
न द्रष्ट्ड़ता नास्तचि दड़्श्यभावःसा ज्ड़म्भते केवल संवदिव ॥

ahaṁmamatvādvyapahāya sarva śrīrājayoge sthiramānasānām ।
na draṣṭṛtā nāsti ca dṛśyabhāvaḥ sā jṛmbhate kevalasavidṁeva ॥

For those firmly established in this *raja yoga*, who have relinquished the states of "I" and "my", no longer is there exclusive identification with objects, nor the act of perception, nor as the one-who-sees. Expansive simultaneity and indivisible sentience truly are the only acquisitions. [The fortress of separateness had resulted in the stress of being penetrated by apparently alien thoughts and suggestions. No longer prisoners in a self-created body, now there are open borders and freely flowing energy].

In modern times, objectless *samādhi* is often mistakenly presented as the only form of *samādhi*. Its purpose is to unite the most subtle aspect of unique individuality to that which is unmanifest and unquantified (it is tempting to call it the "final" *samādhi* in the series, but it is beyond time so the temporal connotation of "finality" does not apply). It must be remembered that each of the steps leading to it are important, they bring about changes in the personal mind and the society around the person. They are ecstatic and adaptive steps, to be honoured and enjoyed.

Referring to the objective *ānanda* and *asmitā samādhi*-s, Gregor says:

> *"...we experience that there is only one self that we all share. Not only do we humans share this one self, but we share it with animals, plants, rivers, geological formations, and the like. The question is then, what is our purpose here? The answer is to be keepers of this garden of Eden, all of us in our own way, and not its destroyers. This is a knowledge that was handed down by all indigenous cultures, and unfortunately it has been lost in all cultures emerging from the so-called sky religions."*[64]

I remember once, a young *yoga* teacher told me of a Buddhist retreat she had just attended, where the teacher had assured them that only rarely do people "attain *samādhi*". She had been told that those special people are monks blessed with the highest *karma*, and that the rest of us ought to modestly work on good behaviour instead, and put off any hopes for the ultimate realisation. Here we see the taint of modern religious history.

Do not make this mistake. You are here to attain *samādhi* **now**. That is the first priority. Good behaviour flows easily from that state. If you are told that you are nothing but an emergent aspect of biology and you need to have your animal urges controlled by law, do not swallow it with credulity. Be a scientist — prove it or disprove it. If the claim is unfalsifiable, it is not a valid claim. Use the one thing that you truly know exists — your persistent witnessing consciousness — to uncover the nature of reality — yourself.

---

[64] Gregor Maehle, "The Relationship between Samadhi and Bhakti", 23rd August 2019, https://chintamaniyoga.com/the-relationship-between-samadhi-and-bhakti

śloka 17

नेत्रे ययोन्मेषनिमेषशून्ये वायुर्यया वर्जितरेचपूरः।
मनश्च संकल्पविकल्पशून्यं मनोन्मनी सा मयि संनिधत्ताम॥

netre yayonmeṣanimeṣaśūnye vāyuryayā varjitarecapūraḥ I
manaśca saṁkalpavikalpaśūnyaṃ manonmanī sā mayi saṁnidhattām II

When opening or closing of the eyes has become inconsequential [due to the collapse of differentiation between internal and external], and the inhalation and exhalation of energy is redundant [due to *prāṇāyāma* engulfing the field to the edges of the universe], then all-encompassing consciousness called *manonmanī* appears, free from bombardment by external diversity and the pretence of separation.

śloka 18

चित्तेन्द्रियाणां चिरनिग्रहेण श्वासप्रचारे समिते यमीन्द्राः।
निवातदीपा इव निश्चलाङ्गाःमनोन्मनीमग्नधियो भवन्ति॥

cittendriyāṇāṃ ciranigraheṇa śvāsapracāre samite yamīndrāḥ I
nivātadīpā iva niścalāṅgāḥ manonmanīmagnadhiyo bhavanti II

When the mind and the senses are thus controlled, for a long time, those of composure, with limbs steady like a sheltered flame, they are immersed in the overflow state of *manonmanī*. [When acceleration and deceleration are no longer occurring, one may be travelling at any high speed and yet feel completely still].

Natural unity

You may not remember right now, but at (or before) birth there was no difference between eyes-open and closed, nor between subconscious and conscious. This most natural *samādhi* is referred to by the term *sahaja.*

In *yoga* we float up to this state by causing the waters to rise. We direct an unusually large flow to the rivers, and the rivers rise until they merge and become a lake. From here, travel between states is lateral and fast. This state is called *manonmanī*, and we desire the inducement of this state in our waking lives. It is an increase in dimension, where the impulse to incessantly compartmentalise, label, and chatter to yourself has been transformed into keen awareness of all that is present. See in an instant all that could ever be said, without saying a word.

It is brain-bending stuff and we need strategies to keep this up. The world of matter is hypnotising. We feel automatic in our tendencies to go after sense desires or indulge fears and insecurities. So, we do an overt daily practice of ascending the mountain and thus expanding our perspective by engaging in the two-stage spiritual cycle. Alternating between states of intense concentration — like a burst of climbing — followed by profound relaxation so that the vista is absorbed. We do this in a *yoga* school where our agency and vulnerability are supported, as in a Mysore style class. Then, the rest of the day has an advantageous tone.

A genuine and sensitive approach is important. It can be tempting to sprint, but sprinting to the top of a mountain might not be what you want. Similarly, resting after every single step could be tedious. We need a balanced mix of active and passive practice, of zeal and rest.

Formal (seated) meditation can also be a tempting object of addiction. Recall the anecdote of the flatmate who would spend 16 hours a day in a closet under the staircase meditating. Even if the fellow was experiencing unadulterated and ecstatic experiences of bliss and truth, it still doesn't seem like an ideal use of a physical body.

śloka 19

उन्मन्यवस्थाधिगिमाय विद्वन उपायमेकं तव निर्दिशामः ।
पश्यन्नुदासीनतया प्रपञ्चं संकल्पमुन्मूलय सावधानः ॥

unmanyavasthādhigamāya vidvan upāyamekaṃ tava nirdiśāmaḥ I
paśyannudāsīnatayā prapañcaṃ saṁkalpamunmūlaya sāvadhānaḥ II

Listen well, those who might attain the status of a high-minded sage! We direct you to the singular method of mastery. Conscientiously apply this method of attention and see *kuṇḍalinī* spin up and dislodge the variety of accreted habits all the way through to eradication/assimilation.

śloka 20

प्रसह्य संकल्पपरंपराणां संभेदने संततसावधानम ।
आलंबनाशादपचीयमानं शनऐः शनऐः शान्तिमुपऐति चेतः ॥

prasahya saṁkalpaparaṁparāṇāṃ saṁbhedane saṁtatasāvadhānam I
ālaṁbanāśādapacīyamānaṃ śanaiḥ śanaiḥ śāntimupaiti cetaḥ II

Having conquered the linear sequence of resolves, having broken their continuity with resolution, the former paradigm [of belief in scarcity born from division] falls away. Gently, gently, the famous "peace from above" shines forth. [Observe creation intently, confront the belief in scarcity, one situation at a time. Do not turn a blind eye, reaffirm your curiosity, and respect all subjects and versions. Feel the rising tide of peace, the inundation of trust, and the outpouring of co-incidence].

Let us skip unsustainable extremism and instead design a spiritual practice that is enjoyable, where you recognise the fountain of vibrancy. There is a reservoir of primordial energy that surges underneath any positive endeavour you participate in. It is something that you can feel to any extent you wish when you are waking or sleeping. It affirms you as a positive agent of will in the world, able to perceive and express yourself far more elaborately and efficiently than using only the spoken word.

Ancient tendencies

We must no longer allow the barrage of sensory phenomena to overwhelm direct perception of the Self that is creating that very same phenomena.

At the start of the spiritual journey, moments of clarity seem occasional, and with persistence they become constant. Along the way you will have circumstances that seem to knock you off the high, positive, and inclusive mental state. Every moment like that is a crucial step where you recognise and embrace fractured tracks or disowned parts of yourself.

Notice conflict and resolve it by inquiring as to how it can serve you. In Mysore style classes you train yourself to do this — perhaps without even realising it. As you practice sun salutations with deep and smooth breathing, you condition yourself to notice knots and discontinuities, and conscientiously breathe through them, creating length and calm. The automatic tendency to see and select positive viewpoints on any subject in any moment is the skill that *yoga* enhances. It is the point of all spiritual practices — skilful action resulting from the union of opposites.

Much of my time is spent with people who have found a path of recognition of the less visible aspects of life and consciousness. Their experience is like reaching up towards the sun, it is as though they found a way to grow very quickly. They become aware of the idea that there might be more, and they attract to themselves people and writings that elucidate methods to move in that direction. Their natural urging towards exploration and innovation leads them to stumble upon great perennial secrets of acceleration. Their attachment to the mundane is gradually loosened, their health improves, and they become nimble and effective.

śloka 21

नश्विासलोप्ऐर्नभ्डि़त्ऐःशरीर्ऐर्नेत्राम्बुज्ऐरर्धनमिीलत्ऐिश्च ।
आवर्भिवन्तीममनस्कमुद्रामालोकयामो मुनपिुंगवानाम ॥

niśvāsalopairnibhṛtaiḥ śarīraiḥ netrāmbujairardhanimīlitaiśca ।
āvirbhavantīmamanaskamudrāmālokayāmo munipuṁgavānām ॥

With the dropping of the breath, with the stilling of the body, and the partially closed, lotus-like eyes, the ideal form [of the snake-like spine and quiescent breath] comes into view. This is the manifesting seal of *amanaska*, [where the senses that are turned simultaneously in and out, the supramental state,] for those most eminent among sages [who may roam the entire sky of imagination, with pleasure, as a *khecarī*].

śloka 22

अमी यमीन्द्राःसहजामनस्कादहं ममत्वे शथिलिायमाने ।
मनोतगिं मारुतव्ड़त्तशिून्यं गच्छन्तभिावं गगनावशेषम ॥

amī yamīndrāḥ sahajāmanaskādahaṃ mamatve śithilāyamāne ।
manotigaṃ mārutavṛttiśūnyaṃ gacchanti bhāvaṃ gaganāvaśeṣam ॥

The great ones, the best of the ascetics [those known as *kṣapaṇaka*, who have uprooted love and hate, dissolved the subject-object-verb relationship into pure knowingness, and are naked like the sky], have a naturally occurring *amanaska*, and a loosened notion of identity, conceit, and attachment. For those, the play of neurosis and the whirls of compulsivity become null. They rest in the essential *ākāśa*, the sky-of-the-sky.

Some time is spent by these students experiencing euphoria and epiphany, a sense of knowing and understanding that transcends ordinary mental machinations. With the secure groundwork of *āsana*, these episodes can come in hefty waves without knocking them over, and without the chasms that one might expect when a psychedelic experience is artificially induced. At times a quickening occurs. Each step up the mountain results in an exponential increase in yield. The further up, the greater the reward. This is in contrast to the diminishing returns that occur with drugs.

As people spiral upwards, the loving nature of the individual combined with their sheer excitement of the discovery make them want to tell their friends and family all about it. Often, these early attempts result in a series of disastrous disappointments. The student realises they are unable to describe the states and experiences, and a feeling of futility comes. The wind is knocked out of the sails and the elated state itself seems to decline.

When it returns, it can seem to have become adulterated by material reality, the reactions of others having affected the initial purity. There is an unrequited desire to have others also stretch upwards, perhaps a feeling of guilt or obligation or loneliness. It also can be jarring to realise that sense gratification, financial accomplishment, and social positioning seem no longer to be the pinnacle of human affairs.

There can be such despair that one may want to get off this path of acceleration. The noble aspirant may try to bend themselves back to the previous level, to act normally.

Sometimes a student is successful in this — you can stop doing *yoga*, you can resume alcohol consumption and shopping, you can abort the process to an extent[65]. Many, however, having seen what they saw, must continue — even if it means letting go of past comforts, social cohesion, familiar friends and pastimes.

---

[65] Modern Indian and "new age" ideas, being quite linear, would say that you resume the journey from this point, in a subsequent incarnation. This is a distortion that nonetheless can be helpful, for a while.

śloka 23

नविर्तयन्तीं नखिलिन्द्रयिाणि प्रिवर्तयन्तीं परमात्मयोगम ।
संवन्मियीं तां सहजामनस्कां कदा गमष्यिामि गितान्यभावः ॥

nivartayantīṃ nikhilendriyāṇi pravartayantīṃ paramātmayogam I
saṁvinmayīṃ tāṃ sahajāmanaskāṃ kadā gamiṣyāmi gatānyabhāvaḥ II

When all of the senses and their associations have left, I will proceed with *kuṇḍalinī* [and her forceful swoon] to union with the total Self [via my notorious trance of visibility]. I go with her [as the rivers overflow in all directions, overwhelming existing channels], superseding the previous states, to the original knowingness [where physical senses are supplanted by non-instrumental perception and I am omnidirectional, secure and pleased, with thunder and light accompanying great upliftment].

śloka 24

प्रत्यग्वमिर्शातशियेन पुंसां प्राचीनगन्धेषु पलायतिेषु ।
प्रादुर्भवेत्काचदिजाड्यनद्रिा प्रपञ्चचन्तिां परविर्जयन्ती ॥

pratyagvimarśātiśayena puṁsāṃ prācīnagandheṣu palāyiteṣu I
prādurbhavetkācidajāḍyanidrā prapañcacintāṃ parivarjayantī II

With high quality explicit examination, one crushes and grinds the ancient tendencies until even their aroma is gone. When diffuse thought activity has been overcome, one may thus ride upon an active form of visionary sleep, called *yoga nidrā*. [Attend to the conditions of consciousness at times of turmoil to reveal the voice of truth, always ready to be heard above the violent reactions of the material].

The gift you give

In a way, we are all alone all of the time. As we have seen, the only thing that we can be logically certain exists is our universally large Self and the figments we create, sometimes taking the form of objects and others. Many times we must face this paradoxical realisation.

The end goal of *yoga* is indeed a state known as *kaivalya*, stemming from the same Sanskrit root that is used in *kevala kumbhaka*. It signifies one whole spontaneous state without an auxiliary. It is isolation in the ever-present and infinite Self. You are all that is, that is all you are.

Any resistance to being alone must thus be transformed, as must our tendency to judge or invalidate the paths of others. The compulsion to change people or have them adopt our views is actually an effort to avoid feeling alone. You do not need validation from others, and you do not need a tribe of followers to support your view.

Typically, loneliness is solved by the validating presence of another. A warm and generous smile affirms your existence. It gives you assurance that you are worthy of another's attention, eye contact, and time. The willingness of another to engage and accommodate you warms your heart and you validate them back in kind. It is the provision of ease.

You can give yourself this gift more directly. After all, everyone loves giving and receiving presents. You can give the gift of warm and patient acceptance to anything, including yourself. If you want the person you see in the mirror to smile, you wouldn't try and poke at the glass — you would change the source of the reflection, and smile yourself. If you want happiness in your town rather than acrimony, you must start it yourself.

Be benevolent, acknowledge and attend to the physical entity that you pretend is you, and the physical forms that you pretend are other people. When you wish for things in the apparent external world of effects to change, change yourself first. In doing so you are changing the phenomenal world.

śloka 25

वच्छिन्निसंकल्पवकिल्पमूले नश्शेिषनर्मूिलतिकर्मजाले ।
नरिन्तराभ्यासनतिान्तभद्रा सा जृम्भते योगनियोिगनद्रिा ॥

vicchinnasaṁkalpavikalpamūle niḥśeṣanirmūlitakarmajāle ।
nirantarābhyāsanitāntabhadrā sā jṛmbhate yogini yoganidrā ॥

All kinds of mentality, intentional and distracted, are thus interrupted, and the entire web of action-reaction-patterns uprooted, through unrelenting vision. Here, the exemplary one bursts open into the state of unifying quiescence, *samādhi*. [The great simplicity and the great torment, to cognise paradoxical oneness with diversity, is called *acintyabhedābheda*. This view bestows pure and timeless cosmic gifts. Each moment can yield perfect liberation, or utter amnesia. Our personal adventure is to rectify any fixity that interrupts this natural state].

śloka 26

वश्रिान्तमिासाद्य तुरीयतल्पे वश्विाद्यवस्थात्रतियोपरस्थिे ।
संवन्मियीं कामपि सर्वकालं नद्रिां सखे नर्वािश नर्विकिल्पाम ॥

viśrāntimāsādya turīyatalpe viśvādyavasthātritayoparisthe ।
saṃvinmayīṃ kāmapi sarvakālaṃ nidrāṃ sakhe nirviśa nirvikalpām ॥

With this cessation, resting on the bed of *turīya*, the fourth state, above the three ordinary states. Whoever thus, has their consciousness always resting in the powerful female friend, enters and basks in the radiance of the formless. [Periods of *nidrā* increase and the boons from other lives are recalled. In the universe there are many overlapping realities sharing the same space, at the same time, only separated by difference in signature. Shift your tone through your actions, which are manifestations of your intentions, and thus change the effects in your life].

This may be a cliché, but it is also plain physics: what you put out is what you get back. Like frequencies harmonise, they attract and bolster one another. Express the warmth you wish to receive. What is the harm and what is the benefit of wearing a smile 100% of the time?

There is a *mudrā* — an attitude — reflected in the wry, all-knowing smile of the Buddha as depicted in classical art. It is called *amanaska*, and it refers to the state that follows *śāmbhavī mudrā*, where the eyelids are half open and the practitioner sees all forms on the one unified plane.

It can be convenient to pretend that mind and matter exist in separate compartments, with your private mind having no effect on the world. It may be comforting to believe that things inside are less real than things outside, but it is not true. All exists on the same level of reality, all is real. Your thoughts and emotions are forces, and they constantly act upon the world, creating effects. When you act with intention, you project it into the world, striking with invisible force those around you.

When you loosen your personality structure, your sets of beliefs and assumptions, and your tendency to chatter in sentences within your head, you remain fluid and expansive. Notice the word "loosen" here — nothing is lost. Your unique identity persists, you need not fear deletion.

Let go and dive into the ocean. You can allow your surface form to be permeable, you can let empathy and identification with those apparent others occur, feel their feelings and know them to be your own.

As this acceptance, wholeness, and security is felt, you become less concerned with fitting in. Rather than reducing yourself or attempting to drag others in a certain direction, you relax and look in other directions. From this vantage, that had seemed so lonely, you can simply cast the gaze afar and see others who are also accelerated. Many more people, currently living and in other times, can be interacted with. So begins a new kind of euphoric journey, and a different dimension of exploration becomes available.

śloka 27

प्रकाशमाने परमात्मभान्औ नश्यत्यविद्यातमिरि समस्ते ।
अहो बुधा नरि्मलदड्ष्टयोऽपि किञ्चिनि्न पश्यन्ति जगत्समग्रम ॥

prakāśamāne paramātmabhānau naśyatyavidyātimire samaste ।
aho budhā nirmaladṛṣṭayo'pi kiñcinna paśyanti jagatsamagram ॥

While in this lustre of the supreme Self, the darkness of ignorance perishes completely. Those with such shining knowledge have their faculty of vision so occupied with the formless that they do not notice the world! [Augmented vision surges as the conventional senses are impressed with additional information, initially as a vibrating or trembling or flickering].

śloka 28

सदि्धिं तिथावधिमनोवलियां समाध्औ
श्रीश्ऐलश्ऱ्ङ्गकुहरेषु कदोपलप्स्ये ।
गात्रं यदा मम लताःपरविेष्टयन्ति कर्णे यदा
वरिचयन्ति खगाश्च नीडान ॥

siddhiṃ tathāvidhamanovilayāṃ samādhau
śrīśailaśṛṅgakuhareṣu kadopalapsye ।
gātraṃ yadā mama latāḥ pariveṣṭayanti karṇe yadā
viracayanti khagāśca nīḍān ॥

Having finally attained such a style of mind, so very prone to dissolution in the highest samādhi, I take my place in the caves among the clouds at the top of the spiritual mountain. In this arrangement of time-space, my body could well be embraced like creeping vines by the arms of a slender woman, and the singing birds could make their melodious homes in my ears [and still I will be rapt and expansive, unshaken and fully integrated].

Come out of the anaesthetic

A Self-created veil of illusion called *māyā* masks the source of thoughts and material phenomena. In a manner of speaking, we find ourselves blinkered and not able to see past a certain distance. Material objects are so compelling that we forget there is more to be found beyond the obvious. But there is a way to view all in synchronous union, and it is attainable by all, not just mystics or once-in-a-generation physicists.

To see more is to see more of **everything**, more particles and events, an exponential increase in the expanse of vision. This is breathtakingly euphoric. It can be irksome too — to have increasing visibility of negative expressions. But we must allow all phenomena to rise and be transformed according to the desires at play and a sense of timing and scale. Allow all personalities to play and experience ups and downs.

You get to choose the stories in which your form directly participates. Accept all adventures as valid and then select your preferred avenues. By following earnest curiosity and desire in each moment, we skip up the mountain — and by doing so in a publicly brave and passionate manner, we demonstrate an evolutionary way of being.

Lead by example so that all may rise together, by investing energy in the practice, and thus experiencing accelerated and productive joyful circumstances. Demonstrate the process. The definition of morality changes from obedience to rules, to sheer truthful expression of our evolving ideals and commitment to discovery of more of the Self. From the mountaintop, compassion and altruism are obviously joyful and they need no prescription or contrivance.

It ultimately doesn't matter which spiritual philosophies or schools or psychological technologies are used, as long as they are positive — inclusive and uplifting. Select an approach that is experimental and taps into ingenuity. Leave behind the shrinking subservience. Humanity is a species that displays inventiveness and has a great time doing it.

śloka 29

वचिरतु मतरिषा नरि्वकिल्पे समाध्औ
कुचकलशयुगे वा क्ड़्ष्णसारेक्षणानाम ।

चरतु जडमते वा सज्जनानां मते वा
मतकि्ड़्तगुणदोषा मां वभिं न स्पड़्शन्ता ॥

vicaratu matireṣā nirvikalpe samādhau
kucakalaśayuge vā kṛṣṇasārekṣaṇānām ।

caratu jaḍamate vā sajjanānāṃ mate vā
matikṛtaguṇadoṣā māṃ vibhuṃ na spṛśanti ॥

This surface mind may wander, but I am in the highest *samādhi.* At the sight of a pair of pert breasts, or a stunning black antelope, one must comport oneself. From the criticisms and praise of others, be they dull-witted or noble-men, I am far away and out of reach. They do not touch me.

One candle lighting another

Let us continue to accelerate. The intellect can always find a reason to doubt the brightness of the spirit, and just as persistently there is the option to trust and go for it.

Humanity's collective story is of being immersed in materiality so intensely that the non-physical planes are forgotten. This temporary sense of scarcity and lack is followed by recollection and journey back to the broader vision. The duration and tone of the journey depends on our individual predilections. Eventually that which obscures knowledge is removed, while continuing to live a physical life.

The dissolution of illusion on a bespoke path according to our preferences is the high spiritual journey. Individuals come to identify with their narrative and enjoy a unique path up to complete integration.

We have talked about ascending the mountain as though the mountain is an object. But as you do so you will realise that you are the mountain, the mountain is a metaphor for the universe. In fact, you are the witnessing searchlight (subject), the mountain (object), and the interactivity (verb) between them. When these three notions merge together, *yoga* is achieved. Indeed, you are the transmutative flame consuming the whole structure, a dynamism that draws from both the material particles at the base and the spiritual air at the top, joining and unifying in bliss and excitement.

We can do it as a team. One candle can light many candles, as they say, and it is a joy to take intricate turns with others along the way. There are many selves, many mountains of Self, all super-imposed over one another. Each one occupies the same space, sharing all time, energy, and matter. They create local consensus and call it "objective".

All people occupy the same space which is as large as the universe. There is nothing larger than you — you are the size of the universe. I am also as large as the universe — all selves are co-located on the one universal field, superimposed over one another. This is called *svarūpa.*

The physical body of a person is the usual locus of their identity. It is a condensed point in the field, a spark that allows for experiences of separateness. We often identify our centre to be in our head or heart, radiating gradually outward. While all people are really the size of the universe, we create a smaller sphere to play in; like a sandpit, bubble, or garden. The size of the individual radiation, the area they can use as though it is their very own identity, depends on their beliefs. It may be limited to the perimeter of their skin, or it may be larger and more useful.

The preceptor

The notion of an exalted teacher or preceptor is found all through Indian writings. They are often known by the word *guru*. Such a teacher is one who illuminates with a great deal of silence. Silent teaching implies frictionless harmony and the inducement of Self-knowledge. So much peace is present, and things appear to be unmoving, just wavering a little, existing but also not existing, loosely structured — like a fire.

This method of teaching is less about material information transfer and more about sparking and triggering the student to open their mind in a way that facilitates Self-realisations. The words spoken are mere symbols. The student is provoked, in a way, and then lights up. The event that we call "teaching" is of candles sitting near one-another, sharing for a while the eternal knowledge.

I remember watching Gregor Maehle teach once. The feeling was just like observing a fire — watching excitedly as flames of intensity licked against forms within him, and across contributions from the group of people as they tossed combustible ideas into the mix. At times there would be a rapid foment of excitement as the right combination struck and the flames escalated! Everyone was rapturously participating in the experience of uplifting together.

Groups of individual fires become large fires. There is a collective unfolding of individual experience, and a harmonious consumption of phenomenal kindling. In this way, the label of *guru* applies not only to individuals, but also to groups defined by proximity or conceptuality.

The word *guru* itself means heavy, weighty, with gravity, which is reflective of the solid teachings involving many people, exploring the deep and meaningful, all rising together. This is the significance of lineage — it is not for familial or academic pride, and not for externalised power. Lineage is a temporal density, a cortex among many adepts in space.

Even with so much recent translation of ancient Sanskrit texts, we have still only touched the surface of the metaphysical literature stowed away in Indian libraries. It is really only in the 20th century that we began to see a significant volume of translation, with Sir John Woodroffe a notable pioneer. We are at the beginning of Western culture, bolstered by the wisdom of the ancients who saw the need to record things for greater dissemination, rather than teach only their local community.

Everyone moves closer to the spiritual air that is the source and the destination and the medium itself. It induces a glowing life. Experiences that feel like dreams increase as we become comfortable letting go of the old concerns of personality, the old habit of grasping at the membrane of separation. We allow ourselves to notice dreams more often, and we learn to access the dream state while we are awake. The sheer thrill of playing in all worlds at once is the very reason we came here.

As we remember to sit near to our imagination and allow ourselves frictionless ideation, we understand how physical reality is an emanation of that very space. The inclination of humanity is to huddle around the fire as a group, in the spirit of sharing, dancing in the darkness yet staying near the light.

All of us together, honouring the needs of the vast whole, with no delineation between physical, mental, and spiritual bodies. This triple aspect of existence is traditionally represented in several ways, including the three syllables of *aum*, the *praṇava*, as well as the three horizontal lines of the *śiva tilaka*, as shown on right side of this page.

7

How to Teach

"I find this way of teaching to be one of the best mediums through which to approach the intangible, subtle element. The silence. The breath. The moving meditations. Having a framework, a set of sequences, is extremely useful for the majority of students to follow, and within that we provide plenty of openness and freedom. We encourage the students to find their own way to practice. This is what I believe was Krishnamacharya's intention. We are simply providing the tools, the map, and guidance along the way; but ultimately the path the student wants to take to get there is theirs. I see my job as a facilitator to empower people to trust and develop their own intuitive knowing and skilfulness in action."

— *Mark Robberds*

Yoga is expressed by the enthusiastic

As a teacher of Mysore style *yoga*, you simply teach what you know. It is a fluid and spontaneous experience led by the individual students, rather than something scripted in advance.

All you need to do to be a great teacher of *yoga* is to practice it yourself, in a consistent and committed manner for many years — it is that simple. This act of persistent application influences people in many ways, some of which are obvious, and others that are less so. In this way, your personal practice is a paradoxically selfish and selfless gift. Everyone benefits from this self-love.

As a student, you practice and study because you feel enthusiastic. You are so passionate because you keep experiencing more benefits, and this is the unspoken message that you spread, aside from anything spoken.

Remember that you teach *yoga* at all times with your simple presence. You do not necessarily need to go out of your way to spruik it, and certainly there is no need to contrive a special personality cloak. Your personal practice creates behaviours and an energy that is felt by others, and the rest is automatic. Inevitably, someone will ask you about your practice. You have been living life a certain way that radiates outwards, influencing people, and they are naturally attracted to understand more.

You may be called upon to "teach" while working in the corporate sector — a co-worker might ask your advice on something. Perhaps, when you are chatting to people at the beach, caring for your mother, or having a business meeting. You radiate the broader concept of unity and health, and opportunities to share are their own reward.

The traditional method of appointment

Throughout the entire history of *yoga* — up until the last few decades as it has been intensely monetised — the way to become a teacher was to simply practice consistently for a long time, until you were tapped on the shoulder by your teacher. That's it. The person you trust, who helped you get this far, who displays evidence of laudable knowledge and perspective, asks you to help out with something. This is the ideal way to move into the role.

The story of how Krishnamacharya began teaching *yoga* is relevant here. The most intense teachers lived in the Himalayan ranges around India, Nepal, and Tibet. The legend goes that these great teachers who were hidden away in caves had started to notice that even though village populations were growing, there was a diminishing number of disciples that were trekking up to the caves and petitioning to be taught in the traditional way. These reclusive teachers did not usually want more than a handful of students for their entire lives. It was enough to modestly propagate the teachings with accuracy and depth. But the situation was changing, and there was a concern that the teachings would be lost forever. Innovations and new decisions needed to be made.

The normal procedure was for a student to live with their *guru* for some time, called *gurukula*, and when a student has completed their mountain studies the teacher would give their blessing for the student to occupy their own hidden cave sanctuary and also live a reclusive life of austerity and practice. This new teacher would be said to be teaching the lineage of *yoga* handed to them by their teacher.

When Krishnamacharya approached the conclusion of his mountain studies, his *guru* changed the directive. Krishnamacharya was asked to instead re-enter the population, become a householder with a family in a city, and to teach other householders as faithfully as he could. This would enable many more people to be educated.

So, Krishnamacharya's students learned from him while living regular lives. Importantly, their apprenticeships still ran over years of daily study of various ancient texts and techniques that go beyond *āsana*. At the appropriate time, Krishnamacharya would instruct them to teach others.

I was very fortunate to have my original teacher offer me an apprenticeship. For one year, I would "shadow" him on the Mysore floor. He would point out to me what was happening for a student during class — what was directly observable, and other insights. I was eventually allowed to cover his classes when he was out of town.

In the current age, this model of apprenticeship is less common. Now there are "200-hour teacher training courses" that condense selected aspects of *yoga* into a syllabus that is taught in condensed blocks — even as little as three weeks. There are programs that stretch out over one or two years as well, with a greater emphasis on slowly absorbing information and supervised application.

Even without participation in any kind of course or apprenticeship, a personal practice in a Mysore style setting is a very pragmatic way to prepare yourself for eventually teaching with depth and authority that comes from an earnest and disciplined undertaking.

Masters of silence

The greatest *guru*-s illuminate in apparent silence. In contrast to the over-use of language in modern society, there is a potency around the quiet space held by a master teacher. As a member of the audience, as a receptive student, there is a sense that subtle consciousness is being operated, augmented here-and-there by spoken word.

I recall a workshop with the wonderful Richard Freeman; on the first day, when the first session was to start, he just stood there silently. As the minutes rolled on, the chatter of the students also faded to silence. Still, he said nothing. Tiny energetic movements were apparent, waves would build, and you could see he was tempted to catch one and speak. But he waited, again and again, wave after wave, silently, the students in rapture, watching, listening. I don't know how long we were there in that pre-verbal state, but it was almost a shame when we eventually began having a physical discourse and subsequent *yoga* class.

A master teacher invites a student to know by facilitating personal realisation, epiphany, dawning awareness — with a flash of understanding known as *śaktipāt*. This is a far quicker and longer lasting approach compared to delivering verbal or written instruction from one brain to another.

The principle is simple and can be applied by anyone: when communicating abstract concepts, first hold the concept in your own consciousness, contemplate it and remember the unique way it is represented in your subjective experience. Feel comfortable confidence.

After this familiarity is established, allow words to flow naturally. You are now channelling — an image, an ideation, a rich concept. You are describing something that is illumined and nurtured in your own Self.

It is the strength and clarity of the vision that is transmitted, with the words acting as a carrier wave. This is more effective than reading from prepared scripts. Script-based teaching is much less effective — better to speak spontaneously and energetically, while gazing at students, seeking non-verbal feedback, and adjusting the tone and content to suit.

Teaching by example is another method of silent instruction. One mark of a great teacher is an attitude of beaming affection to all-comers. An attitude that integrates stereotypically fiery drive and confidence, along with the ability to rest in resplendent beauty and creativity.

There can be a tendency to worship the messenger. While we may honour various traditions and lineages, the root and primary reason we are there is for the students. The masters do not require adulation. What they want is for us to teach well. We serve the people in front of us.

Our job as teachers is to help these admirable practitioners of *yoga* to be happier in their lives. In each moment, we serve the students and, by extension, the community.

Teaching is a meditation itself

We are the custodians of students' precious time and some of their most raw and vulnerable experiences. They rearrange their lives in order to come to the studio, and we must attend to them genuinely in the spirit of shared growth and aspiration.

As teachers, we curate and attend to the energy of the room. One of the key tools we have is the unspoken receptivity of the students, the mutual consent to open and share a deeper state of being. If we, as space-holders, come to class with a deliberate and considered intention, a sense of balance and brightness, then everyone who attends will rise to that level and maintain it for one another.

A Mysore style teacher ensures the safety of students by keeping a close eye on their movements and by actively engaging with them during practice to identify issues. A teacher delivers education by spotting opportunities for refinement. In class there will be discussion of areas for development, answering questions, and physical adjustments.

We all know how it feels to speak to someone who has their attention divided. Their eyes dart around and they acknowledge you at intervals, rather than a constant connection. A great teacher is a great listener, one who desires unbroken concentration on the subject at hand. Often in class the teacher will operate several simultaneous streams of attention. Additionally, the individuals form a collective personality that can be interacted with. This is all quite a challenge and ought to hold your attention fully for the duration of the class.

On a motorcycle, a rider must learn to maintain an unbroken awareness of vision from both mirrors; who is several cars behind and who is several cars in front; which cars are behaving unpredictably and may therefore stop or turn suddenly; patches of oil or gravel on the road; potholes; which side streets are coming up where there's a risk of cars jumping out across the path; pedestrians and cyclists; lurking police.

Taking on board multiple actors, you project a route through the approaching corner, plot the course that gives you the best combination of safety and efficiency, and are ready to make alterations in real time.

In the same way that a motorcyclist reads the road and maps the safest route in their mind, a Mysore teacher should always know the current state of play in the room, and the next few adjustments they intend to make. They should also have the clarity and awareness to shift the plan as needed.

A Mysore style class is a gestalt entity that can be tuned to an ideal mix of earnestness, exertion, relaxation, and humour. To do this, the teacher must watch and listen to the rate, tone, and volume of breathing, along with non-verbal cues of stress, effort, laxity; people entering and exiting the room, or stopping for any reason.

With this persistent and multi-threaded awareness of the individual and collective energy of the room, a deeply meditative state is cultivated.

What is energy in this context

The content of one's character is perceptible to others in myriad non-obvious ways. This can be explained using mystical language but it need not be. Scientific studies confirm this, and it is also patently obvious — the contents of your mind affect the way you present yourself to the world. Body language, facial expressions, subtle gestures, tones of voice, choice of language, and even pheromones, all contribute to the overall understanding we gain of someone in our proximity. This is commonly referred to as the energy of a person.

People radiate their energetic contents and absorb the same from others as they walk down the street, whether they deliberately interact or not. There is a constant communication on a level that is considered subliminal. This is heightened in *yoga*, and a Mysore style teacher in particular has a great deal of responsibility since people let their guard down in a way that is very different to when they walk down the street.

A class environment might even elicit the most open and vulnerable mood a student permits themselves to ever have, even more than at home. You as the teacher allow them to rest in a space that is permeated by your own energy and the cumulative energy of all the other students.

In Western style led classes, the dynamic is less intimate. It is more like following along with a fitness instructor than being in a school. The students listen to the instructor and enjoy what is presented on that day. In a led class, you must fix your attention on the person leading. You consume the emotional and verbal content on offer. A strong focus must be held on the voice and gestures of the person at the front of the room.

This is in contrast to Mysore style classes where students fix their attention completely on their inner experience, with help on the side from the teacher as needed. It is an interesting middle ground where the student is not completely alone, but is also not lost in a group. The shared space contains friends who have a common investment in getting to know themselves deeply by getting to know the practice.

The initial investment is greater than with led classes where anyone can drop in and follow along. In Mysore style the first few classes are spent being highly dependent on the teacher. Gradually, the sequence is learned and the student can feel more immersed.

Subtle respect

When teaching, there are things to check with regard to your presence. It is wise to pay attention to where you stand in the room, your favourite places and those you avoid. Similarly, notice who you tend to adjust or speak to frequently, and those for whom you have a blind spot. In this way, teaching Mysore style is a potent personal development practice itself, as you learn more about your own attractions and avoidances.

It can be easy to give attention to those who are comfortable asking for it, or those you know well, while students who need help but are perhaps shy or reserved may go unnoticed. As a professional, it is important to give equal attention, verbal or not, to everyone.

As a culture, we are learning more about how to best help people heal through practices such as *yoga*. Trauma-informed *yoga* is becoming more widespread and it is a fascinating window into how to improve your teaching to better accommodate diverse conditions.

When teaching someone with trauma, factors such as remaining in eye-shot and not suddenly changing your location, are very important. So too is modulating your tone of voice and the language you use to be clear and straightforward. Earning trust and consent with physical adjustments is also crucial. There are many insights to be gained here.

We are living in densely populated cities where there is excess noise, rapid mechanical movements, jarring sensations of many kinds, without the natural stress-relieving elements that humans evolved to enjoy like the sounds of birds, feeling sunlight tickling the skin, and opportunities to relax and stretch during the day. While this may not be acute trauma, like being exposed to military combat, it still affects stress hormones.

A pleasant and non-confrontational atmosphere is an invitation for students to slow down and to fully experience each moment in time. Look at the language you use and consider the degree to which you are commanding versus suggesting. Sometimes we definitely do need to command, and sometimes not. People are living in an over-the-top enforcement culture. Traffic police, bosses at work, the bank, and many more actors seek to monitor and catch people. During *yoga* we can cultivate something else.

Yoga is the science of human flourishing, and it is an opportunity for playful self-expression without fear. As space-holders, we are in prime position to help people lift their mood. We can help them trust their sense of personal authority and thus increase their interoceptive abilities and creative vision.

Help students manage ups and downs

In chapter five we discussed the idea of peak performance and the balancing of the two extremes of the nervous system. The sympathetic nervous system can be represented by the Sanskrit term *rajas*, and parasympathetic nervous system activation is labelled *tamas*.

When Ashtanga Vinyasa Yoga is practiced in a Mysore style environment, students increase their interoceptive ability and thus notice the state of *rajas* and *tamas* within themselves more effectively, moment to moment. Such awareness helps them remain balanced in the centre of the two, and this poise is called the state of *sattva*.

As a teacher, you assist by observing and reflecting. When someone is moving into over-amplification of the sympathetic nervous system and displays stubborn traits or mechanically driven pushing, you notice it and assist them. Similarly, if someone is resting a great deal and shows apathy or an inability to lift their energy levels, so too you can help.

An approach favouring *rajas* can be seen on a broad level too, where unyielding strictness is seen as a virtue. This is often observed in Ashtanga Vinyasa Yoga. Sometimes, injury is even seen as a badge of honour in the pursuit of perfection, a necessary rite of passage. This approach will please many people, and many people feel they **require** this — they thirst for a severe level of authority and will not be sufficiently motivated by anything else.

Such focus on precision and mastery is a true and valid way to practice. The idea is that with perfect concentration and a humbly gradual approach to each posture, injury would never occur. Sharath Jois, has said as much — that the greatest cause of injury is a lapse in concentration[66]. It happens when you drop your focus, or take too many liberties — move too quickly through the postures, decide to tackle poses that are beyond your reach, or deviate from the precise breath count. This is an effective method of practice that errs on the side of *rajas*.

A primary goal of the practice is to flow through all of the poses and transitions, *vinyāsa*, without becoming distracted or feeling the need to pause, rest, or otherwise break the flow of breath and movement. The series exactly the same number of total breaths every time they practice.

This yields formidable physical and psychic stamina — stunning emotional resilience is developed. There are many times in daily life when the mood drops, when tones of defeat or victimhood can creep in. When the *āsana* regimen of orthodox Ashtanga Vinyasa Yoga is practiced well, it spreads into all other spheres of life. It is the spiritual transformation, beyond mere relaxation. It spurs positive imagination and makes the mood automatically lift through Pavlovian conditioning.

Discipline is a limited expression of something far greater — enthusiasm! A *yogin* may rise before the sun every morning to do their practice, and this can look like discipline at times, but it is in the spirit of a play date, an agreement to create sparks of interest using an obligation-free tool that we have been given by cherished elders[67].

---

[66] Conference Notes, Mysore, October 2014

[67] This view of discipline has been expressed by many, including J. Krishnamurti in an interview during February 1974 and Julia Cameron in *The Artist's Way* (New York: TarcherPerigee, 1992).

But the strict approach is not suitable for all people at all times in life. A balanced and generous *yoga* teacher must be willing to teach people who have already tempered their perfectionism, or who have had enough injury in their lives and have learned the lessons that a bloody-minded approach has to offer. People young and old frequently need a safe space to restore their bodies, and true community spirit is reflected in a class format that embraces everyone.

Similarly, a balanced teacher will recommend exercises and therapies which suit the needs of the individual, regardless of whether they can be incorporated into the *yoga* practice or not. Climbing, cycling, bushwalking, and many more things are a part of humanity that bolster spirituality and *āsana* alike.

I live in a small coastal city where surfing is a popular pastime. Many times, our students will balance their *āsana* with at least as much time spent in the ocean. In the ocean they are relaxed, operating on a rhythm much larger than their own. Such connection with the expanse of nature seeps into their consciousness and helps neutralise the spiky tension of the city's artifices and mechanisms. They tend to err on the side of calm; during their practice they allow *tamas* to counteract *rajas*.

To be honest, I'd been practicing for several years before I personally saw the kind of toxic zealotry I had heard about in *yoga*. Stories of crazed behaviour from cults and religions are renowned through history, but I had heard from teachers a generation older than me about international *yoga* culture having its fair share of violence, mindless ritualism, and bullying. When these teachers would tell me the stories, it was so far from personal experience in my home town on the coast of Australia, I assumed it must have been since eradicated, or maybe it was an American thing!

Eventually I met people who desired an all-or-nothing approach — where the literality of the teachings is considered gospel and no variance shall be brooked. A sort of flagellation (of self and others).

It was a shock to see, and I am glad I do not see it any more. Such an approach is hard to sustain, and in my limited experience, such an extremist must either double-down and become even more violently committed over time, or at some point abandon the system altogether and then demonise and advocate against it. A large part of my intention with this book is to show that this is never how *yoga* was meant to be taught, it is an unusual interpretation of *tapas*[68].

Regardless of age and approach, a healthy level of fire is certainly needed, and this is the meaning of the term *tapas*. It is a commitment to expedient progress, taking the form of regular practice and deliberate conscious effort in every part of the process.

I certainly enjoyed throwing all of my energy at the practice in the early years, erring on the side of injurious behaviour, eagerly pursuing the goal. I don't quite remember what that goal was, but I certainly felt like I was going after it with all I had. At some point, discipline began to look more like masochistic insensitivity, and I re-evaluated my approach.

There was a very pointed moment when I finally succeeded in performing a pose after struggling physically and mentally with it for months. "Yes! Finally! About time!" I thought to myself. Then, mere seconds later, my beautiful teacher Dan, in perfect timing, began to tell me about the next impossible pose I would be asked to accomplish. It really sank in that day — this will never end! There will always be another cycle of challenging exertion eventually followed by the elation of success.

I realised I could temper the harshness of the exertion phase, give myself a more pleasant experience, with less sweat, swearing, and daily anticipatory loathing. This perspective proliferated through my life outside of practice as well.

---

[68] Sharath related a similar point of view in a conference. He said some people think *tapas* is military strictness, being hard on yourself. He said it really means being consistent, maintaining a suitable lifestyle, avoiding excessive sleep, food, and the like.

An experienced teacher, who has "been there and done that", will be able to assist students to transform their urgency into a smoother distribution of energy through time, through parts of the body, and through modes of *yoga* being practiced[69]. This task is easily accomplished when we use the method of Krishnamacharya, which became known as Mysore style[70].

In the one room you can have fiery students being firmly scolded for allowing their concentration to wander for a moment, practicing alongside retirees who do not require that approach. With this sort of well-rounded group dynamic, each segment draws support from the other.

Individuals dancing on sacred ground

The artistry of teaching is in delivering just enough information. Recall the idea of a master teacher imparting insights silently. How this is to be done, what methods to use — much of this cannot be stated in a book. There is a need for teachers to be taught extensively by great teachers. They come in many forms and contexts, so you may find yourself bringing teaching techniques from all manner of influences. Our teaching style is influenced by our whole lives, and we feel gratitude for the opportunity to creatively express ourselves.

I have never taught anyone anything. They have all figured it out for themselves — I merely provide a safe space and ample encouragement and enough hints for them to accomplish their self-discovery.

---

[69] Craig Procter learned from masters like Shandoor Remete and Robert Lucas, and he apprenticed under veteran Australian teacher Eileen Hall, learning the advanced series alongside some of the most famous teachers of the 21st century. On the topic of how practice changes over the decades he told me: *"The more I practice the more I see what releases the body, nervous system, mind, and gland secretions. Reducing the amount of āsana I need to practice creates a more efficient practice [straight to the point]. In the end you need to see why you're doing it. What I was taught is it's about long head and shoulder stand and or prāṇāyāma. How much strength do you need for them, what type of strength does it take on one hand, on the other hand flexibility, brings [the release of energies, gland secretions, lightness, easy, bliss]. You can hold shoulder stand or head stand in bliss for one hour so the poles in the body get reversed. It's easy to find bliss through extreme āsana but the older you get the more you pull on refinement to find it."*

[70] TRS Sharma (speech delivered in Mysore, February 2020)

Persistently keep this question in mind: why are we doing this? Is it to seek approval, or to meet the guidelines of a distant tradition, to ameliorate some kind of insecurity, to create a sense of certainty in an uncertain world? Teachers must be able to explain the reason for their instructions, and "because that's the tradition" is an insufficient answer.

We are individuals dancing on sacred ground. We have a baseline system and lineage that we teach, and yet each individual student and each teacher works together in the moment to express spontaneity. Any rules of *yoga* are the jumping-off point from which to explore our bodies and experiences. We harness and enjoy the system — we rest on and refer to it, but are not caged by it.

Excavation through time

Another interesting result of regular practice is a vivid experience of travelling through time, through one's own life. This is particularly pronounced when the student begins *yoga* in middle-age. There are so many pieces of accumulated tension and fragments of injury, and they come to the surface, bringing along memories of historical incidents.

It tends to be the case that recent issues in the body appear and are resolved first, and then eventually contact is made with injuries or imbalances from the distant past. It is desirable to have a teacher with expertise and the willingness to customise practices to help individuals work through their needs as they arise.

Equally important is the need for students to be vocal in their felt experiences and their needs. A relationship needs to be cultivated through communication and earned trust. It cannot be overstated that teachers must actively encourage people to reveal their bodily twinges as their practice progresses — it is vital to help them understand that pain is not something that needs to be stoically endured.

The tendency to keep pain — perceived as failures or blemishes — secret until reaching a breaking point is very common. It is perhaps an effect of a culture imbued with authoritarianism and the habit of suppressing one's true desires. People feel like the struggle to try and get their needs met while meeting the obligations of society is an unavoidable part of life. Advertising plays on guilt and fear of not being good enough as you are, as if authority figures are waiting to catch you making mistakes.

Sometimes this carries over into *yoga*. It can be exhibited through the over-willingness to "suffer in silence", to "just get on with it", to have an all-or-nothing approach, to suppress or hide pain. You can see how this trait would impact the planet too — the tendency to ignore warning signs (pain) and keep on slogging through using the old methods, even when things seem dire.

As a culture we are realising that it is our birthright to have radiantly healthy bodies, that physical culture is not an extravagance — it is actually a high virtue.

Institutions of varying kinds are all too willing to make declarations about social virtue, and decide what is right and wrong. In *yoga* it is simply emphasised that abundance is the natural state, and that a belief in scarcity and the manufacturing of fear and guilt are the only true "evils".

Common sense approach

When a student suffers an injury, there must be a customisation of the practice to address it. After all, we have the benefit of time and space to look more closely at our bodies and make educated decisions.

Any injury can be transformed into an educational event. It would be a mistake to hold onto traditional guidelines as immoveable commandments — the very definition of dogma. As we discussed earlier, it is witnessed in increasing measure when a school degrades, whenever tradition is permitted to reign over common sense. Veteran teachers around the world state clearly: it is always a valid option to skip or modify a pose.

Yoga gets easier in the long term — the trick is to get through the first few years without burning yourself out, or creating unnecessary drama. Observe a practitioner of Ashtanga Vinyasa Yoga with multiple decades of daily practice under their belt. They are lithe, there is an almost alien sense of effortlessness. We can all get to that place if we pace ourselves, develop interoception, and allow the fascia to remodel gradually.

Hamstrings

The most common injury seen in *yoga* is a hamstring strain. Sometimes this is provoked purely by *āsana*, but often other sporting pursuits of the student, in particular running, sprinting, and kicking, contribute to the situation. The likelihood is increased by factors such as shortened muscle length, poor posture, and excessive neural muscle tension (when nerves become stuck and do not slide and glide as much as they should)[71].

---

[71] Liu et al., "Injury rate, mechanism, and risk factors of hamstring strain injuries in sports: A review of the literature," Journal of Sport and Health Science, Vol. 1, Sep 2012

In the case of hamstring strain, regardless of the causes, a good physiotherapist will ask the student to stop stretching the hamstrings and instead focus on strengthening them. This can be done in the Mysore style environment by removing or modifying the forward bending poses, and adding in helpful poses that would not otherwise be found in the primary series. After some time, the student will be able to cautiously re-introduce forward bends, and continue practicing the traditional series, having rehabilitated their body in the shared studio space. All the while, they have kept enjoying the community bonding qualities of the studio space.

Lives are enhanced by this approach. The student might have otherwise felt like abandoning the practice, or that they should stay at home until healed, or keep pushing through pain in a way that prevents recovery.

Shoulders

Another common injury in *yoga* is a strain of the shoulders related to the push-up movement performed during sun salutations and jump-backs. These movements are repeated so often that general tension can build, and if there is any underlying weakness or insufficiency of technique, problems can emerge.

A good teacher will teach the fundamentals well, and spot incorrect technique early, before injury occurs. Nonetheless, injury still can occur. In these cases, in addition to strengthening drills, it can be beneficial to offer radically different ways of achieving the desired effects of sun salutations and jump-backs.

In chapter four we looked at key reasons for practicing *sūrya namaskāra*: to perform a deep breath cycle similar to *bhastrikā prāṇāyāma*, to overwhelm the downward facing tendency of the material mindset, to stretch and reset the spine in preparation for the next pose, to engage in an act of trailblazing positivity and playfulness, to psychically connect to our breath and silently affirm our existence beyond the mundane.

Clearly, doing push-ups is not an essential part of this. A favourite way to substitute a traditional jump-back is to:

1. from seated, roll backwards and forwards a few times
2. kick up into shoulder-stand without using hands for support
3. hold yourself there for a moment, engaging legs and abdomen
4. with control roll back down onto your back
5. perform bridge or fish pose, lifting up with a deep inhale
6. roll back down on the exhale
7. bring knees into chest without using the hands
8. roll up into a seated position, ready for the next pose

Here, we have performed a plyometric exercise that involves a full engagement of spinal stabiliser muscles — the intrinsic core, as well as an extension and flexion of the spine. Along with this, a deep breath cycle, all without using the shoulders — giving them a little break.

Spinal extension

A notable aspect of the primary series is that it features many forward bends and not many back-bends. This is for a good reason — this sequence is intended as a preparation for the more balanced intermediate series. Remember that the primary series is *yoga cikitsā* — literally "*yoga* therapy". It recommends a **temporary** focus on rehabilitating the body from much chair-sitting and sedentary lifestyles.

It addresses the fundamentals of being able to lift ourselves up off the floor using our upper body, and being able to bend over, squat, and sit on the floor with ease. This is quite a basic function of the human body, but it can be lacking in varying degrees depending on the person.

Eventually, after a period of building a healthy foundation using the forward-fold-dominant primary series, it becomes necessary to build on this and give the body more backbends. Backbends are poses that extend the hips and roll the shoulders back and stretch the abdomen and inflate the chest. It is at this point that we start introducing poses from the second series — the intermediate series.

Inclusive yoga

Do you want a studio that caters for a special subset of the human race, or do you want to offer *yoga* to anyone who expresses an interest?

This is a crucial question to ask! People who start *yoga* over the age of 50 are perfect students for Mysore style *yoga*. Often their spirituality is well-refined through the normal experiences of life, and they need an *āsana* practice that will fortify their efforts. Why not also make it easy for people with diverse needs and non-normative bodies to attend class?

It is prudent to interview prospective students and get an idea of where they are in their lives, their limitations, how frequently they can attend, and then work on helping them experience the depth of *yoga*. Perhaps by electrifying their lives with a strict form of *āsana*, but there are many other approaches that may be more suitable.

Are you able to do this? Are you able to adjust the teachings to suit people, or are you only able to teach one syllabus within strictly policed parameters? It is very reasonable for a young teacher to teach exactly what their teacher taught them, but as they gain experience, it is reasonable to expect a teacher to stretch their capacity to serve. The two-stage spiritual process is visible here as well: a narrow focus on a highly specific set of parameters to the exclusion of all others, followed by an expansive perspective that welcomes all.

It is okay to have a specialised studio that caters to people who want the strict and intense method of practice that is prominent in modern memory. This approach is appealing to many and is valid in its own right. There is a notorious style that features teachers who are unyielding in their critical eye and sharp words, or who perform strong physical adjustments that are sometimes injurious yet are romanticised as a kind of "opening". This is suitable for some, for a while. But as time rolls on, those who continue to practice inevitably find a more accommodating approach to be beneficial.

It is a wonderful thing to have a flourishing studio that caters to the fierce students as well the other, more therapeutically-oriented groups. You can absolutely have students who thirst for firm discipline and need to earn validation practicing **right alongside** those who have different physical capacities and priorities in life.

It is quite a scene — to have a 25-year-old, who thrives on being treated firmly, pushing and exerting themselves in earnest, practicing next to a white-haired lady who is more concerned about maintaining rotator cuff integrity so that she can be a better babysitter for her granddaughter.

The beautiful truth of the matter is that there is in the world a far greater number of people practicing customised versions of the traditional sequences than those who practice to the letter of the law. There are many adaptive Mysore style environments all around the world that radiate love and inclusivity and which facilitate this approach. Unfortunately, it is also often the case that people find themselves unable to practice anywhere but at home. This is either through sheer absence of teachers, or a lack of teachers willing to be flexible in their approach.

The trope of a *yoga* teacher as a disciplinarian has been overplayed, as has the stereotype of a person with a monk haircut, detached and bland, telling people to subdue their desire and strive for peaceful passivity. The suppression of passion that this projected persona necessitates can lead to distorted behaviours out of public view, such as bullying and predatory inclinations. The discovery of these by devotees can be shocking and cause them to lose their way. Often these people have done wonderful things for their students and the world, and yet they slip into deplorable behaviour. All kinds of degradations are possible. A life-long commitment to the path is required. A serious teacher must continually eradicate negative tendencies through the practice of dissociation from superficial addictions and aversions. They must cultivate intense concentration on the highest possible ideals.

The practice of *yoga* fills one up with vigorous energy, and this carries responsibility. Even when one has previously demonstrated virtuous deeds, they are still able to forget, turn their back on the source of the energy, and slip into material gratification and addiction once more.

Śaṅkara notes an obstacle to successful practice is "the tasting of joy"[72]. This refers to the potential for distraction by increased pleasure in worldly activities — which ironically have been boosted by practice. By all means, enjoy the benefits accrued, but beware excess.

It is up to us to create the role of a modern *yoga* teacher. The existence of creeps and abusers does not mean that we stop teaching in a way that is emotionally intimate. We must not create distance or passivity out of fear. We must be more active, willing to engage, equipped with lessons and cautionary tales, and new ideas to improve our teaching.

When I look around the studio, I see discipline there in spades — students are already willing to make financial and lifestyle arrangements just to be able to come. They are already willing to go through intense physical and emotional experiences during the practice.

The support we offer frequently takes the form of exuberant encouragement to put in more effort, but also often it is on the other end of the scale. The granting of permission to ease up, take more time, go gently, skip things that are hurting, or even abbreviate the practice so as to meditate for longer or to perform relaxed and easy stretches.

The lesson that all multi-decade *yoga* practitioners have for us is that you can be more focused on ease than you might initially think. Consistency of practice is much more important than pushing intensely in any particular pose. A practice with enthusiasm and patience is what brings the outcomes you desire — it just takes a little while.

---

[72] Aparokṣānubhūti *śloka* 128

Outreach

In stepping into the role of teacher, we need to completely embody a caring practitioner, eagerly awaiting any opportunity to share and assist with infectious enthusiasm. Create courses, provide guided meditations, workshops, reach out to people, write articles, be an advocate of the spiritual life, be active in elevating people and fostering harmony.

Mysore style *yoga* is an introverted practice, and at times it can appear aloof or nonchalant, even arrogant. As we have seen, spirituality can be a cloak to enable one's desire to escape the world, or to justify a certain violence or nihilism. We counter this by fostering positive community, facilitating bright conversations before, during, and after practice. Teachers have a duty of care to proactively reach out to students and regularly remind them that pain is not a compulsory part of the practice and that they are welcome to share concerns and questions.

Student #1

Here is an email I once received from a student that shows just how close to breaking point people will linger before revealing their pain.

> *"I've been really struggling with my neck/upper back recently, and I think my practice may actually be making it much worse. When I had a four week break due to a holiday and moving house, my neck was great. It felt normal for the first time in over a year.*
>
> *When I restarted my practice last week, my neck was bad again, really bad. I think the headstand and some backbends are aggravating it, so I'm trialling stopping the primary series when I get to the end of the seated sequence, but even that's still aggravating it.*
>
> *I'm not sure what to do, I don't want to give up the practice but I may have to accept the fact that what I currently do is not good for my neck. I'm not sure whether to push through, modify my practice, look at other styles, or even give up yoga, which I really don't want to do as it has given me so much. Sorry for the ramble, do you have any suggestions?"*

You can sense the despair and frustration in this message. This student kept this struggle to themselves, burying their pain, for months before this point of finally opening up. If it wasn't for the relationship between student and teacher, including pro-active communication outside the studio, this student might have abandoned *yoga*, or scaled it back.

In this case we worked with a physiotherapist to diagnose the issue — instability and weakness in the cervical spine — and incorporated the prescribed rehabilitation exercises into his *āsana* practice. This ensured the exercises would be done diligently, to the physiotherapist's delight.

A short time later the pain and despair were resolved. It took several months before certain poses were able to be practiced, as the student explored deeper sensations in the body, in a safe environment, learning to understand subtle sensations of fatigue and strength.

The student continues to enjoy an exciting and motivating practice and has a greater appreciation for learning their own anatomy. Crucially, he learned that things which may seem like certain defeats are always surmountable, and that early discussion is helpful.

Student #2

A 27-year-old man who had become paraplegic 20 months earlier due to an eight-story fall, made enquiries about practicing *yoga*. He initially contacted us asking about Western style led classes, but I advised him that Mysore style classes are the most suitable. We met the following day an hour before the afternoon Mysore session was to start — as I often do with new students. We chatted to determine the scope of his restrictions, the progress he had been making, and the existing rehabilitation and fitness efforts in his schedule. He had already improved enough to be free of a wheelchair and be able to walk around reasonably well. One of his legs was rather functional and the other much less so, nonetheless the situation was improving, and there was every reason to assume it would continue.

We developed a practice based on the themes of the primary series — spinal extension and flexion, with deep breathing, followed by standing and seated poses to stretch the back and sides of the body, followed by a closing sequence. Every week we would catch up for half an hour before class to go through his sequence and remove things that had become too easy and add new challenges. For the first few weeks much of the work was done on hands and knees, or on fists and knees, as one wrist was not able to extend completely. We placed a lot of emphasis on deep breathing and experimentation.

He was not fazed by being in a room full of people doing more advanced poses. Not even for a second did he show any nervousness around what others might think. He was oblivious to the notion of embarrassment and was very excited by the environment and what it might provide him. It reminded me of when I walked into my first Mysore class.

In time, he began being able to do *sūrya namaskāra* in a way that is pretty close to "traditional Ashtanga". He can now do the standing poses reasonably well; he can balance okay. The seated postures are where his progress accelerates most, he spends several minutes in each forward fold as he can feel that the volume of time spent directly relates to the benefit attained. His back and hamstrings are becoming more elastic as the fascia releases. The spasticity in his right foot is easing and he is noticing greater mobility and co-ordination.

After three weeks of *yoga*, **he was able to stop using opiate pain relief** for the first time in 20 months. He has not used them since. In the kitchen at home, when he is preparing meals, he can pivot from side-to-side gracefully. Advanced postures may be out of reach for him. But who knows? He keeps improving. An innovative and non-dogmatic approach is essential. It is satisfying to facilitate and a wonderful thing for other students to witness.

Note that we really did not heal him. Neither did *yoga*. Living in Australia, with a good healthcare system, he has access to various neuro and physio therapy experts. But most importantly, he possesses a strong personal drive to develop himself as far as he can. He is eager to push for more information, to question the conservative prognosis offered by the medical field, and to politely decline the sympathies of well-wishers when they entice him to abandon hope.

Where is the sense in excluding people because they are not thin or bendy enough? Can you imagine saying "no" to a request for help, on the grounds that you are not willing to modify a sequence of poses?

Student #3

Recently a woman in her 70s started *yoga* with us — her husband bought her a class pass as a Christmas gift. Together they have been exploring ideas around healthy living in a way that was either not available or seen as fringe only a few decades ago. They are discovering the joys of improving their diet and exploring physical culture, embracing their retirement years by learning how to better themselves and develop their capacities.

We established a routine of about a dozen poses, divided into sets of three postures, which she repeats a few times each. Each trio serves the purpose of sections of the primary series. There is a set of poses that perform the functions of *sūrya namaskar*, then another set of standing poses, floor poses, and so on. This is very much the style of Krishnamacharya as expounded by Śrīvatsa Ramaswami, mentioned in chapter three.

After a couple of months of *yoga*, aside from having a newly buoyant gait, she told me that she loved being able now to reach the top shelves more easily in the kitchen.

And the others

There are so many more stories of people finding the studio and enjoying their progression to liberation. As has been discussed, some find themselves fitting into a standard model of the traditional sequences and methods, and others benefit from a broader approach.

Scorching hot practices, intense body modification, exalted spiritual epiphany resulting in trembling rapture! All of these things are seen on a regular basis, yet just as often is a pragmatic and even understated evolution of health.

We are all in increasingly fortunate positions. The understanding and communication of the benefits of good health spread by various physical culture movements in the past 50 years are beginning to have an effect.

The stories my grandfather used to tell of his life in middle age were a fascinating time capsule. *Yoga* was not an option in those days, and the idea of exploring athleticism outside the realm of competitive sports was a rare luxury. The idea of athletic and spiritual enjoyment being a primary focus in life was deemed unrealistic, even irresponsible. The focus was on survival and having a large family. When he retired, he could have begun a physical culture regime with zeal, having a sizeable pension and accumulated savings, but it was not very common; no-one was talking about it. So, for no good reason, his weight increased an awful lot, resulting in his mobility dropping, and by the time he died at age 94, he was glad to exit.

With every decade that passes, we find ourselves more conversant in matters of health, and each generation that pops up finds themselves less willing to wave the white flag and give in to morbid beliefs around ageing.

The Sanskrit led primary

The Mysore style format is self-paced and geared to allow you as much time as you need on each posture each day. It is possible, however, that the overall pace of your practice might gradually wane and even verge on subdued. To manage this, there is traditionally a strong led class held weekly in a Mysore style studio.

This special class is taught in the Sanskrit language with a challenging tempo and a minimum of alignment cues. It is a metronomic calling out of the primary series postures and transitions. It is like a weekly examination of your abilities. In theory, everyone in the class takes precisely the same number of breaths. The idea is to practice at a consistent rhythm, executing each pose with minimum of fuss, possessing sufficient stamina to maintain that pace for the entire time.

Where there is a population of advanced students, a led intermediate series class can also be held, an astounding display indeed! In the suburb of Gokulam, in the city of Mysore, people would gather in the waiting room of the school — the *śālā* — to peek at the advanced students, bending and floating with such athleticism.

The proper path for most people is to learn *yoga* in the Mysore style format and to eventually be able to attend the weekly led class. People who are progressing well but have not yet completed the primary series can still attend, they simply stop once the class has reached their normal finishing point. They pause there and wait for the closing sequence to commence so they can re-join and complete the class.

For advanced students who have moved well beyond the primary series this is a nostalgic and enjoyable activity that grounds them and ensures their current practice does not come at the cost of the fundamentals.

Teaching as a lifestyle

For the first few years of my life teaching *yoga*, having quit my corporate IT career, I only taught led classes — around 20 classes per week at gyms and Western style studios. For years I felt sheer joy every day at not having to work at a desk, or to suffer through endless meetings, to drive a car long distances, or to write reports and plans for things only vaguely linked to some kind of positive benefit to people.

My job now was to wake up in the morning, get on my bicycle, ride to practice in the Mysore style studio that I would years later take over, drink coffee in the sun, teach warm-hearted people at gyms, apprentice with my teacher, and sit in the sun some more. I felt wealthy for the first time in my life, even though my income had just dropped dramatically.

The time spent in a salaried career helped me a lot for years to come. It showed me that I can dig deep and work and commute 70 hours a week. I developed a strong work ethic and inner resilience. Teaching deeper *yoga* is about subtle forms of demonstration and relationship. If you can show a practical approach without jargon or loaded new age words (even the word "spiritual" can be problematic), you will be doing a good service to busy people who are juggling a career and parental duties.

Sacrificing some sense-gratification in order to develop your practice also sets a good example. If your desire to help people leads you to teach without charging money, again this is a powerful example to set. You **can** afford to do this, to devote yourself. You cannot afford to be half-hearted. Give teachings to those in need.

People do all kinds of heroic things in the name of romantic love — so expand this trait and do things that benefit others out of the intense love that arises from awareness of the Self and all of the figments within it. Allow your actions to span generations, the broader world community, and the planet. The idea is somewhat like gambling, betting the house, going all-in. The gesture is profound — we invest ourselves fully into ourselves, and the most valuable thing we have to invest is our time and energy.

As teachers we exude our innate qualities and attract students so aligned. If you have a steadfast and disciplined approach, the students who identify with that approach will be drawn to you. They will thrive on your timeliness, devotion, and the glow cultivated by your personal practice. They will model the ideals they see like moths to the flame. If, on the other hand, your behaviour reflects a practice that is unstable or inconsistent, you will attract students with the same inconsistency.

Your job is to use any techniques you can find to help people cultivate earnest dedication, to make the most of this opportunity and move beyond short term thinking, momentary discomfort, and inertia. There are many ways to spur motivation and discipline[73]. Ultimately, anything that works in the moment will do, and it will often change over time. The surface mind must be compelled to acknowledge and remember that there is

[73] Bhagavad Gītā 4.25 – 4.33 mentions a few classical examples: *karma, jñāna* etc

indeed something beyond it. That is, the all-encompassing Self spanning all time-frames and objects. It is the aspect beyond pettiness, it is wise and generous, able to see the big picture.

All of these ideas are intended to stoke *bhāvana* — the fervent "calling into existence" of that which ignites us. With *bhāvana* you can accomplish anything. It flows with an urgency that overwhelms doubt and second-guessing, it impels your greatest expressions of character. An automatic turning upwards of perspective in each moment, an ingrained habit of automatically noticing phenomena in the world that are best-suited to those highest ideals — which have also become your strongest desires.

Sustainable teaching

The secret of sustainable teaching is to get out of the way. You did not invent *yoga*; you are just passing it on. You don't have to come up with unique content. The concept of breathing deeply and stretching your chest and having a nice introspective experience stands on its own. Don't get in the way with any misplaced feelings of authorship. Hold space for the students and help them help themselves.

The teacher merely manages the fire, stoking and adding material, intervening occasionally. The fire is self-sustainable for the most part. An initial ignition is often needed, but be under no illusions: it is the effort of the individual that matters.

When students come up to you after class, watch how you receive the compliments they give. The compliment is not really for you — even if they believe it is. The truth is that they have generated their own positive experience through their practice, loosening their own restrictions and increasing awareness of their higher Self. You may have played an important part of the process, but don't mistake the words coming from your mouth as the thing that had the positive impact on the student.

It is the *yoga* itself that has had the impact, you are just the vehicle that delivered it. Your job is to be a competent messenger.

You should receive compliments well by reflecting positive energy back to the person. Graciously thank them, and then direct their awareness to their own virtues. Highlight their efforts, point out something they did well in that class. Thank them for coming and for allowing you to enjoy your part in their positive experience.

Get out of the way and let people practice so that they feel empowered and free. To interfere with this natural process by contriving your own special program of poses will consume your energy. If you fall into a belief that you are the one who delivers the good feelings to students, you will suffer a co-dependence. It is not about you. You can make it about you and your separate self if you want to, and that behaviour is common at the moment in a pop-*yoga* market. I remember once, an instructor confiding in me on the situation they had found themselves in. Their students expected "creative new flows" from them, every week, new variety and stimulation, and this had been happening for years. The teacher told me she regretted having "made a rod for her own back."

I did this for a while too. I was personally practicing Ashtanga Vinyasa Yoga in a Mysore style setting, but I was teaching a more popularist style at gyms. It was fine, but it felt disingenuous. I was benefiting so much from the effects of a set-sequence, and yet here I was teaching something that I had realised was limiting. The joys of inner exploration caused by the more traditional practice became so great that I felt I was depriving people of something.

Eventually the feeling of dissonance increased in me to the point that I decided to try teaching what I practice. So, rather than invent new combinations of poses and transitions, I began to just teach a simplified version of the primary series each class. I would remove a few things to make it shorter, and maybe add in a couple of poses or shuffle things in the seated section. I still do this if I teach a led class at a commercial studio. About 80% is static and 20% is a spontaneous selection of the other poses from the primary and intermediate series.

I employed this consistent approach for a year and class attendance was not affected. No-one commented. Everything was fine and I got to witness people getting much better at *yoga* much more quickly.

After a year of emphasising the same sequence I did an experiment — I taught a *vinyāsa*-flow-variety class, just like the early days. Well, I tried anyway! Within a few minutes the quizzical looks and feeling of mild annoyance from students was too much to bear, the unspoken message was: "stop whatever you're doing and let us do our practice."

Allow people time to dissolve

When students enter the classroom, their energy is affected by things they have done that day, and their life in general. For example, say eight people walk into your afternoon class — two have arrived early to chat amongst themselves, one has come in exhausted from a long night shift, one comes in feeling anxious about a meeting scheduled at work.

Imagine that people have a sphere of energy around them, and the size and content of the sphere changes depending on their health, emotions, and experiences each day. When they do *yoga*, this circle expands and becomes more harmonious and attractive. Positive states of acceptance and optimism are induced by breathing deeply and stretching the chest.

Through the process of *yoga*, the energies people bring to a class will merge, and the negative ones will dissipate while the positive increase. The principles of love and trust that *yoga* seems to create are actually native to conscious beings. They do not need to be cultivated, rather, they re-emerge when surface noise is allowed to become quiet.

The overarching gift that a teacher of Mysore style *yoga* offers is a warm and supportive presence. If nothing else, you just need to stand there watching. People will be reassured that their safety is being monitored, that their general technique is being checked, and that they are emotionally held by someone who is giving them their exclusive attention. It might feel weird initially, just standing there observing… as they bend and stretch… but that is the role!

If you can give your presence for one or two hours or however long their practice is — then you might become one of the most important people in their lives. You will be a guide that they look back on as having been there for them at pivotal moments. You can positively influence them in a way that does not happen in many other contexts as an adult. Our society can really make people feel quite small and undeserving. To have a supporter, a backer, holding space for them is often their true need.

Here is a chance for your personality to expand into a new realm. Introverts are often said to be the best teachers; they tend to start slowly and gradually blossom. Be brave, don't slink back into the shadows, treat this as a privilege, and step into the spotlight a little bit at a time.

One more thing

Sometimes, despite best efforts from everyone involved, someone will bow out of Mysore style *yoga*. Even when taught as a rehabilitation practice to fortify one's body and lungs as they age, there is an aspect that cannot be escaped: it increases self-intimacy.

I am grateful to have had people share their reasons for stopping the quiet, self-directed Mysore style practice. I have been told: "I prefer to just switch off", "I find it hard to not be competitive", "I feel too lonely".

Ashtanga Vinyasa Yoga can be the easiest or the most difficult form of *yoga*, depending on your approach. It can serve you for 100 years, or you can burn out in one week.

This is a long-term project spanning multiple decades and all occurs in perfect timing. The thousand heads of Patanjali as depicted in mythology represents that there is a unique path of discovery for each human, and we are honoured to be involved where appropriate.

8

THE PLACE TO BE

We have discussed several facets of the spiritual process and the ascent to the mountaintop. The practice (*sādhana*) consists of alternating between varying forms of concerted effort (*abhyāsa*) and expansive relaxation (*vairāgya*). The intent is to climb in a rhythmic and natural fashion according to our own sense of joyful play and appropriate timing.

The practice is implemented through *āsana*, *prāṇāyāma*, and techniques like *trāṭaka* and *śāmbhavī mudrā*, which reduce exclusive identification with the coarse aspects of physical reality. Students of this method attain increasingly easy access to states of absorption (*laya*) and super-concentration (*samādhi*). This delivers the enhanced ability to view and interact with all aspects of reality, from the very subtle to the obvious.

Mysore style *yoga* encourages practice right up to this pinnacle. This format allows us to go beyond physical fitness, and **far beyond** merely feeling "better than before".

Mysore style allows for a sense of immersion that was previously only found in ashrams and caves by those who were willing to go without societal integration. It provides a means to sustain an evolving practice while expressing passion and commitment in life.

We have discussed the function of limitation and filtering, how the surface mind experiences tiny increments of time and space, and creates dialogue in the head that narrates experience. The veil of *maya* is our consensual amnesia, the deliberate forgetting of the vastness of reality for the purpose of experiencing things as if for the first time.

We looked at the antidote to cynicism called *bhāvana* — the dizzying delight that is provoked through fervent application. This is a crucial ingredient on the upward journey to the top of the mountain, where we find the greatest concentration of bliss called *ānanda*. This essence accompanies the naturally passionate and visionary state of existence, and it is only obscured by the tendency to judge, which in turn compels attraction and aversion — be it conscious or habitual.

The topic of desire is clouded in modern spiritual culture. What people typically call desire is but an initial spark of enthusiasm immediately covered by layers of doubt and guilt from generations of suppression. A person's typical experience of desire is heavily tainted and frequently causes them pain. Desire is thus seen as a problem to be eradicated, but **conditioning** is actually the problem. It is a mistake to restrict desire, although the intellect finds it rational to do so.

Desire is fuel, and it is supposed to be experienced in greater measure as sensitivity is increased and inner authority is trusted. Along the way, beliefs are brought to the present awareness for review and adjustment.

The innocent experience of desire without modification is so wonderfully euphoric that it alone makes life ecstatic and beautiful. Our birthright can thus be reclaimed when the guilt of religion, the fear of reverting to animality, and myth of scarcity are abandoned.

We looked at methods of subtle attention. Interoception points to our perception of physical components beneath the skin — such as the heart and fascia. So too the forms of meditative absorption recommended by *yoga* that draw us deeper into the ever-present originating consciousness, via the imagination, with its fast-moving stream of forms that are often only viewed by adults when sleeping. Dreams are always occurring, all of the time, and we have seen techniques that help us pay attention to them while awake.

We discussed the attitude that emerges with the realisation that all things, whether thought of as internal or external, actually exist on our screen of consciousness. The logical conclusion is that positive service and attention expressed to others is actually a gift of service and attention given to figments within ourselves, and is always a good idea.

The practice of Ashtanga Vinyasa Yoga has been explored, along with the typical experience of students across the primary, intermediate, and advanced series of postures. They optimise the nervous system and invoke the untapped inner energy called *kuṇḍalinī*, by means of *āsana*, *prāṇāyāma*, and *bhāvana*.

We have explored advanced *āsana* practice as a form of spiritual demonstration. As omnidirectional beings we show how one may stand firm as a pillar of society while also resting in perceptive states and behaving with generosity and efficiency.

A natural extension of this is to move into the role of teacher. As studious practitioners themselves, people can act as conductors of energy, and teach *yoga* in a variety of environments. Great teachers demonstrate the process of releasing the formerly compulsory attachment to materiality, and showing a positive life with integration of all levels of existence.

It is time to look at a meditation to bring it all together.

Your life as a narration

The Sanskrit word *asmitā* means "(the sense of) I-am" and it is the apparatus that focuses consciousness into something specific. It provides the ability to describe, allocate, and categorise. It is the masculine counterpart to the feminine *maya*. Without this partnership, the present moment would have an overwhelming amount of content.

With *asmitā*, the notion of personal identity sprouts. The unified being splits into "I am this, you are that. I am me, doing this, with that". Rather than all events and all places existing as one integrated whole, *asmitā* creates a sharp focus on individual events consisting of moments and objects. The function of *asmitā* reliably maintains the illusion of boundaries by ignoring most of the other co-located objects in existence.

The topology of the mountain is such that we have increasingly expansive awareness of connections and options at the top, and isolated definitions at the bottom. We have inklings, intentions, and ideas up high, and decisions, instances, and sentences down below. The mountain is our entire world and *asmitā* is the point on the face of mountain from which we carve a path and tell a story.

Human life is thus a story of the changing position of "I am" as it moves down into narrow awareness and up into broad awareness. Our position changes as much or as little as we desire in each moment. The spiritual journey is one of noticing when we are hypnotised by the material world (when "I am" is lower), and when we feel a greater sense of knowledge and free will (when it is higher).

From an elevated position we see more and understand more. It is possible, with practice, to jump in and fully live in the world with purpose while retaining the knowledge that we are playing a game of amnesia. We can learn to skilfully operate the *asmitā* function, enjoy the illusion, and remember to return to the top when excursions are finished.

Western culture has a strong bias towards the bottom of the mountain. Society has become productivity centric and materialistic. Being able to complete tasks with great efficiency is lauded and rewarded. Wandering about in the imagination is not. Modern cultures have largely forgotten about the need to interrupt the downward motion of *asmitā* and view the **causal**[74] ingredients up high.

The surface mind has been mistakenly given credit for all of the things our species creates. The filtering component of the brain, that part of us that reduces the scope of attention, has been appointed king!

Turn around and look up the mountain

It is spectacularly easy to remedy, in theory — just pause, turn around, and look up the mountain. Close your eyes and look at the images. The nature of focused attention is to "go" where-ever you look, to identify with what you are observing. **So, invest attention upwards.**

It's effortless to be addicted to material things, and it's also effortless to be addicted to your full and true Self that contains everything. If you are tired of identifying exclusively with the material, then look elsewhere. With a simple reorientation, the material world is seen in context.

Sometimes material content will seem more flat, as though there is more space between it and you. It is by means of this increased space that the rest of reality can make its way into your regular conscious experience. The material world is an ephemeral projection on a field, and there is much to be found in between the observer and the material world.

Note that seeing the world as forms on a field of imagination does not mean maligning or discarding it — you just play with it in a different way. This is discussed by many great teachers. It is said that an established *yogin* who is

[74] The plane where causes are found (also called the "causal body") is equal to the *vijñānamaya kośa* of the *pañca kośa* model shown in chapter five and the *paśyantī* level of speech (*vāc*) in chapter three.

situated in transcendence sees all the objects of the material world as equal in essence[75]. Be they rocks or gold, all have the same value.

Śaṅkara famously refers to cultivating the same attitude to all objects of the material world that one would have to the droppings of a crow[76]. Objects are effects, they come **from** spirit, from the substrate. We desire to be jolted out of the hypnotism of linearity, and such acerbic vigour from the spiritual masters can be helpful.

Sometimes strong measures must be taken to loosen the grip of exclusive attachment to material objects, fuelled by the dopamine kick of task-oriented activity, and the tendency to find stasis comfortable — even when it is unhealthy. The coarse intellect has declared imagination to be unreal! The surface mind is bound to the world of material effects. It operates in one straight line, excluding the riches surrounding it, and it is famously difficult to interrupt once it has found itself in control.

Adepts please! Do remember that the assumptions of materialism are arbitrary conveniences. There is no solidity. The body is made of energy and is being permeated by waves of cosmic energy of varying frequencies as though it is made of vapour. The world you see, the world you pretend is solid and that you play within, is in your imagination. All objects are apparitions — **and** they are quite real! Everything is real, existing in your imagination. Your imagination is **the only thing** that you know is real.

Imagination seems to be infinitely large too — it never runs out of space. Every time you see something new, there is space for it in your imagination. It accommodates the droppings of a crow, the trees by the river, history, religion, politics, motorbikes, comets, your friends and family, popular culture, and theories of multiverses and simulations. All of these things are equal, they have the same level of real existence, and we seek to disrupt the mistaken perception that any one thing is more or less valid than another.

---

[75] Bhagavad Gītā 6.8

[76] Aparokṣānubhūti *śloka* 4

Wilful self-rattling

In this vein, it is well-known that disruptive events "happen to us" from time-to-time, and they often seem rather negative. Earthquakes, pandemics, accidents, tragedies all serve the purpose of jolting the superficial personality out of its bubble of limitation, its monotonous sphere of attachments. These events can be frightening and inconvenient, even devastating, nonetheless there is a purpose served.

Many times, people will relate that they made very important changes in their lives as a result of injury, death, relationship breakdowns and such. Sometimes an incident forces a course of action that had not been taken due to the inertia of routine.

One can adopt a more pro-active position of "wilful self-rattling". Once you understand the tendency to cover over the uncertainty of reality with mundane routine, you may then counter this by performing deliberate and conscious disruption. It is uncomfortable to the half of you that seeks permanence, the doubting part of you that presents worst case scenarios, but when you discover that there is another half of you that relishes and **requires** the unknown, there can be harmonious fusion of your two sides.

Predictably, there is a word in Sanskrit for wild mystical rattling. It is *avadhūta*, and is used to refer to a philosopher or ascetic who shakes free, kindles, or agitates. *Yoga* advocates using the body, breath, and manipulation of energy to disrupt stasis, sometimes taking students to the edge of physical comfort. It can feel like fainting — intoxicating and visceral — expressed with the word *mūrcchā*, meaning to "swoon". Euphoric and positive clear vision unfolds as the creative hemisphere leads the intellect by the hand into the forest of amazement.

Life can be like this, like when you were a child and every day was a brand new adventure. You were unhampered by adult routine, residing naturally at the mountaintop, and you can be there again — this time possessing the additional benefit of experience in material affairs. The very word ecstasy means "outside of stasis". It can be as simple as taking a holiday somewhere new, or driving to work a different way, or stretching the body to a position it has never experienced before.

Lucid waking

The point of this whole endeavour is to **wake up into the imagination**. To light up the dreaming state and the waking state at the same time, and to be aware of their interactivity. High up the mountain, above particles, sentences, and isolated moments, consciousness has a free-form quality. There, we become skilled navigators of supervisory states.

Lacking this awareness is to be orphaned from the total reality — stuck at the material level, oblivious to the functionality of the spiritual sky. No wonder there is such fear in material existence — people are playing in the dark. Realise that the dream scape is operating at all times, it was there before the body was born. Upon it flows a constant cavalcade of forms, and it can be viewed at the same time as the sensory world.

Day dreaming is an easy way to access this window. Knowledge can be transferred to the physical brain through this medium. Dreams seep rich multidimensional concepts into segmented sequential reality.

Seated meditation is a prime method of bridging worlds. To meditate, you must slow down and sit still. When you do this for a period, you slip outside of movement and time. Rest in the underlying awareness of your spatial playground where time is indistinct. By entering this space, you will see the relationship between dimensions of yourself.

Of these adventures, people often remember only vague images and chaotic events. Beware concluding from this that dreams are unimportant — this would be a faulty application of logic based on a narrow scope of attention. Pay attention to your full Self. Don't lock parts of yourself away; bring the unconscious into the light. Your dreams are there to be enjoyed and to act as informants. Neglect, suppression, and denial are the wickedness we seek to overturn.

This is the home stretch of a long game. We have been hypnotised by the giddy thrill of things appearing separate and thus new, shiny, and pleasurable. Our attention has been fixed on everyday situations to the extent that we have forgotten the bulk of reality. We have created a society that rewards us for operating within strict parameters, and it both subtly and bluntly dissuades us from breaching them. Nonetheless, we can remember the start of it all and live with total awareness. This may mean branching out from dominant culture, and using that momentum to explore other paths.

Mountain dynamics

The Sanskrit word *pratyaya* is used to refer to the nebulous ingredients in consciousness — non-verbal moods, aspirations, ideas, thought forms, geometric analogies, proto-linguistic poetry, musical metaphor, memories, and interesting visual constructions. (Note this is a different word to the well-known sense withdrawal called *pratyāhāra*).

Yoga helps us notice *pratyaya* of varying kinds. They range from the mysterious intangible notions that slip through the fingers, through to ordinary mental content and verbiage.

This gradation is reflected in common psychological models such as the hierarchy of needs. These modern ideas draw greatly from the Indian *cakra* (also spelled *chakra*) schema for categorising contents of consciousness. In the *cakra*-s down low, we find expressions that are concerned with survival, scarcity, and short-term material needs.

As we proceed up the mountain, up the *cakra*-s, the *pratyaya* are found to be generous, social, and altruistic. At the very highest *cakra*, they are ethereal and less contingent on time and space — persistent and independent, existing apart from any specific person, ready to be identified and employed.

The practice of *cakra* meditation is to habituate the stopping of chatter[77] and other low *cakra* activities, and instead map the higher spatial terrain. High level *pratyaya* are available there to be increased, decreased, or sent forth into the world via physical activity.

We must learn to keep this cloud of immaterial ingredients in our day-to-day experience, and we can develop this skill during *āsana* practice. A Mysore style environment offers a place to work on seeing the material world and the causal world of ingredients at once. We learn to glide between partially formed events without slipping into distraction or sleep. We retain reality in its nebulous form, like molten gold that can easily become forged into the shape of a ring.

Keep the fire lit, resist the temptation to solidify or limit the view.

The surface mind is intrinsically uncomfortable with flux. It seeks illusory permanence, and it is all too willing to reduce the scope of consciousness in order to pretend that there is certainty. **Stay molten**[78].

---

[77] Aparokṣānubhūti *śloka* 108-110

[78] Here there is a pertinent analogy with the physical body. Stay flexible. Just as materialists deny the spirit, so many spiritual people deny the body. You should put your legs behind your head! Or be working consistently and gently toward this kind of outcome, where the joints of the body bend deeply in equal parts flexion and extension. It matters a great deal. If physical flourishing is skipped over, then the unification of opposites promoted by *yoga* as a spiritual method, is incomplete. For a *yogin*, the body is a joyous thing. Peaceful, yes, but brimming with energy and more exciting than the most awesome temple — a place of celebration that you don't want to leave. Materialism is essentially a death cult, where all members agree and reaffirm to each other that physical capacities diminish after a certain age and that death then becomes a blessed relief. Anyone who claims to feel more physically able as they age is met with ire. It is often those who are most imprisoned who will offer the greatest resistance to being freed. Years ago, when the benefits of a shorter working week were being uncovered by psychologists and economists, I found it was those most ravaged by underemployment and inequitable labour conditions who were the most vehemently dismissive of the notion that society could evolve in such a way that people can work less and be healthier and more prosperous.

Keep persistent awareness of the whole of consciousness even while acting in the world. Śaṅkara says that this is the real mindfulness — to always consider all planes as part of your one true Self, in each moment[79]. When you do so, the joy and bliss that we encounter in physical sleep streams into your waking reality.

Keep noticing it. What do you hear right now? Do you hear the sounds of the non-physical, or is ordinary content consuming your attention? Do you feel the ecstasy of uncertainty, or are you encumbered by solidity? As strange as it sounds, this is the way to expand. This is the meditation on *nāda* referred to in Yoga Tārāvalī, the absorptive focus on vibration itself as perceived in consciousness. It may take the form of sound, vision, proximity, mood — all sorts of words point roughly to these phenomena.

The personality, the intellect, the surface mind, must come to understand that it is a subset of a greater scope of knowledge, and it must consent to cooperate. It must agree on its own rational terms to release the stranglehold so that it can enjoy a more diverse stream of ideas and therefore a greater benefit and an expanded identity.

The fabled spiritual enlightenment is a consequence of such expansive identity. It is the revelation of natural, self-generated bliss and knowledge that arises instantly any time it is called[80].

Look for it

If you wish to speed things up, imagine there is a reservoir bearing down on you, a drip feed waiting to be opened, and you control the tap. When we resist this fluidity and work to maintain stasis by pushing desire away, we slow down evolution. Instead, open the tap through action in the highest spirit, following your genuine sense of curiosity, interest, fascination, and excitation — and allow experiences to flow.

---

[79] Aparokṣānubhūti *śloka* 122

[80] Aparokṣānubhūti *śloka* 125 - 126

The experience of excitement is a present sensing of the future, and intellectual musings are a commentary of the past. The time delay between an initial excitation and the subsequent dialogue is often minuscule, nonetheless it is still always after the fact. The reasoning mind follows experiences and thereby receives evidence of its progenitor.

The most foundational *pratyaya*, right up the top of the mountain, at the highest *cakra* where all the rivers meet at a point in the sky, is reflected as positive expectancy, genuine interest, innocent curiosity, and unconditional love. It is the word "yes". Follow the course of action indicated by the charge of your psychic sense.

But what would happen if everyone just did whatever they want? Many people do! They are called children. And while they need a little bit of protection and support, their growth occurs from direct experimentation. They evolve their own parameters. You do not need to over-condition them or replace their adventurous spirit with dull life administration.

Self-directed inspired action is a self-correcting strategy. If a person has a buoyant attitude and a respect for their own inner authority while performing misguided actions, they are acting in a more useful fashion than if they were to do the intellectually or societally-determined "right" thing, out of obligation, with a loathsome attitude. If what you really want to do is "bad", non-optimal, destructive — you will quickly receive feedback from your world. You will have followed your sense of earnest truth and you will learn the lessons you need. Your sensibility will evolve while keeping the tap of self-respecting energy open.

Your compass will improve faster this way. You will merge the intensity of joyful exploration with the values you come to appreciate, and also any physical laws that become apparent.

Nothing happens without the pursuit of joy. There is no use in going down an intellectually virtuous path that lacks excitation and curiosity. One might even say it is an immoral act — self-denigrating.

Stop slouching. Sit up tall and open your chest. Take your cue from the natural world. Imagine if a flower was afraid to blossom, or the bees sat around analysing their wings and wondering if they could fly, but not daring to try? This gift of analytical intellect is meant to augment, not restrict, our natural activity. It operates best as a narrator, rather than an arbiter of action or judge of morality.

There is no prejudice, doubt, or guilt in the natural world. If you enjoy the gifts of your own Self more fully and freely, then you will find yourself content, not tempted to steal the gifts of another, or of the ecosystem. It is logical and moral to develop your passion and cheer. This is the difference highlighted in the Indian texts between *kāma*, pleasure derived under the assumption of materiality and separateness, and *ānanda*, the intoxicating pleasure that is recognised while situated in the unified Self[81], *ātman*, where diversity and singularity co-exist.

Play your song and let it blend with the songs around you. The habit of arguing with or silently recoiling at the unpreferred aspects of the world must be addressed. If not, our expansion grinds to a halt. The unflinching willingness to see all things as equal is called *samadarśin*[82]. We apply this equanimity, and then we apply *viveka* — our power of preference.

At every step we have ultimate power to choose the intentions we carry, the *pratyaya* we hold, and what aspects of physical affairs we give our energy to. Even though others may be intentionally negative, we remain in every moment aware of the choice to extract from every situation a positive result. No matter the perceived intentions of others, the most rational thing you can do is to kindle awareness of your own will, intention, vision. It quickly becomes an automatic experience of play, harmony, and serendipity.

Unconditional love is unconditional permissiveness; if you will not permit a part of another person to exist, then you disown a part of yourself and maintain a boundary. If you see suffering and corruption in the world, you

---

[81] Narada Bhakti Sutras *śloka* 6 - 7

[82] Bhagavad Gītā 5.18

must consider it as valid, yet unpreferred[83]. Strangely enough, the suffering and corruption you see is a part of your very own Self, now made visible in the external world, to be used as fuel.

You can transform powerful negatives through equally powerful positive action. Activism is ideally fuelled by rushes of clarity and clear declaration of your needs. State your position using your intention, your words, and your actions. Anger arising from witnessing injustice can be powerfully constructive[84]. Perhaps you will receive the exciting idea that you can use your privilege to advocate for people around the community.

You must have constant access to your own assertiveness and confidence. A flower asserts itself strongly as soil temperatures rise and hormones in the water it receives trigger its bloom, literally called "budbreak". Be in the habit of acting on your will and breaking out of passivity.

This is *yoga* — to acknowledge, integrate, and then construct reality. Be willing to see and reconcile **everything simultaneously** — the preferred and the unpreferred, pleasure and pain, imagination and material effects. See like this, and then choose the way you want it to be. Define your unique human experience this way.

Do the things that give you the purest sense of enthusiasm and you will align yourself with the concept of magical guidance. Remember that intention permeates time, sweeping into the future, while intellect and dialogue are in the "past".

[83] Narada Bhakti Sutras *śloka* 11

[84] It is important to know that pure momentary anger is a valuable event when experienced naturally and in good faith. It is a rush of alignment, an instantaneous knowledge of what you do and do not want. Other behaviours commonly associated with anger such as malice, manipulation, regret, and violence are unfortunate effects of suppression. True spiritual anger is revelatory and lasts only a few seconds. The same is true for laughter and crying, they are all extremely clarifying when treated as informants; they present problems only when twisted into distorted behaviour tainted by rumination and conditioning.

Tones influence probabilities

A unified being enjoys physicality in the richest ways possible, so relax and smell the roses. Act as though all will be revealed at the right time — act with the assumption of positivity. This is the true view of spiritual gratitude and contentment. Every single crumb, every granule of circumstance in the material world can be found to serve.

Notice the *pratyaya* that is active in any moment. Such feeling-tones are interpreted very personally and rely on your inner language and symbolism[85]. Invite mysterious feelings of "gravity" to keep tapping you on the shoulder, independent of any self-talk. Know that in addition to noticing them, you can actively select and fashion them to suit your needs.

I use a local mechanic to service my crummy old car, he is in his late 70s and is an interesting bloke to talk to. One day I asked him for advice on a problem with my car. As he took a look, he remarked that he was supposed to have had double knee replacement surgery so that he could bend down more easily to fix cars. Lamentably, with the coronavirus lockdowns his surgery had been delayed.

A couple of months later, I dropped in to see him again. I had not been able to fix the car myself so I thought I would leave it for him to have a closer look at. When I dropped it off, he suggested we go for a short drive together so that he could experience the issue first hand. As he was driving, I noticed that he was struggling a little to press the clutch pedal, and I said to him "Jeez you really need to get that knee surgery done". He said to me "Oh I had it done two days ago, it's a bit sore".

---

[85] There is a tone that is native to you, it is present when you are awake and asleep, and you will recall experiencing it when you were a child. It is your natural and indescribable signature and it lay within all of your actions, just as gold is within jewellery (refer to Aparokṣānubhūti *śloka* 22).

I was surprised, "Really?! You're back at work already?". He said "Yeah they wanted me to stay in hospital for a week and then have a month off work, but I told them I won't do that and demanded they release me." He seemed to be bounding around the workshop chirpily, a far cry from what I would have expected.

He continued, "You know, I really feel that you have to interact with the body as though it is a separate entity which accumulates beliefs based on your behaviour. I felt that I should just get to work and act as though the healing is swift and proceeding well, rather than being bedridden, and my body will take that cue and heal quickly."

I was dumbstruck. I didn't realise he had such views! It is always nice when someone older, well distanced from any new age claptrap, reveals such transcendent ideas.

Our invisible intentions accompany our actions, regardless of whether they are conscious or automatic. They co-mingle with our mundane physical actions in the world and they play a crucial role in shaping outcomes. That placebo effect won't go away, as much as we may ignore it. You tend to get the result that you anticipate.

Trust that **you are supposed to feel good all the time**. Who put the idea in your head that life is a mixed blessing? At the very least, trust that **you deserve to** feel happy. Having a rollicking good time while you traverse the merry adventures of life is an absolutely natural way to exist. There is a certain arrogance required here, a brazen willingness to interrogate the paradigm you find yourself operating within, and then create alternatives.

Lead with the vision

The greater the practice of *yoga*, the greater the capacity to sculpt in this way. When the processes are honed, mere minutes, even seconds, can be enough to elevate your vision for productive and joyous experiences.

How do you do this in a practical sense in a busy world? To answer this, note a crucial aspect of breath and *āsana* that Gregor has mentioned:

> *"The breath leads the movement. Rather than movement following and responding to the breath, the breath should initiate the movement. By prioritising this way, we will be moved by the breath like the autumn wind picking up leaves."*[86]

It is advised to initiate *āsana* by means of the breath — to begin a breath before beginning a physical movement. In the same way, it is advised to initiate other physical actions in the world using the imagination first. Rather than moods and abstract states of mind **following** the physical events of the world, instead set and reset the intention **before** acting.

Before you do something, hold a statement like "I am wholly positive and reflexively loving, and I easily see how events in the world serve me and deliver a life of excitement". Decide that all situations and all actions are for positive benefit, and then act like that is the case.

Face the truth that all things occurring in your world are influenced by your intentions, for your benefit and the benefit of others. You are the consciousness that all is played upon.

The only person that can judge you is you. All words, whether they come from inside your skull or from the mouths of others, are located on the field of consciousness that is the Self.

---

[86] Maehle, G., "Ashtanga Yoga Practice and Philosophy" (Crabbes Creek: Kaivalya Publications 2006)

Take advantage of the instants in life that seem to provoke disruption and nudge elevation — where we find our perspective suddenly altered, in a flow state, or a state of greater understanding and inspiration. Such experiences break us out of the spell of mechanical living and lift us into a perspective of greater clarity.

A young student related a story of moving from a regional area to a big city. He is studying music, and already actively composing and recording in his bedroom. When planning for the move, the idea occurred that he could busk for money. That idea excited him and also gave rise to a natural fear of performing publicly. What followed is an expansive experience of conscious creation. His family had a firm belief that he should get a proper job in advance so as to afford rent. But he wanted a certain situation that was not compatible with security of employment. He allowed himself to feel an interesting weight on his shoulders, a sense of needing to go to a specific place of discomfort, putting aside the concerns of family. He permitted a situation of unemployment to exist for a little while and it meant he had no choice but to busk. This turned out to be a vital growth process for him.

This is an example of having intense *pratyaya* in the conscious experience, a peculiar sense of nervous excitement, followed by a commentary of fear and reasoning around the need to secure the illusion of safety in the form of employment. He chose to allow the exciting *pratyaya* of spontaneity and the energy of uncertainty to stay active and fuel him.

Rather than subdue his anxiety through rationalisation, he instead sculpted it into its twin sibling — brazen willingness. He added to the mix the *pratyaya* of trust, and oriented himself in the direction of open possibilities rather than the comfortable narrowing of options.

He could have missed out on gaining those first experiences of live performance on the street and had his growth delayed. But he found a way to embrace and advance the moods and feelings. He could have waited for a calamity down the track to rouse him into overdue action, as is so often the case for people in middle age. But he made use of mild discomfort, got on the front foot, and assigned his own meaning.

These moments are available to us at all times, but we are not usually aware of just how often we distract ourselves from the urgency and uncertainty of life. So many edifices we create to soothe us, to distract us, and to keep us looking at things down the mountain.

It might be tempting to think that this sort of freedom and spontaneity is easier to manage when you're young and childless. Maybe — but we know that life is anything but solid, and anything can happen any time. So many good things pass us by because we're busy being comfortable. The more we get used to the feeling of instability, the more we can seize the gift of dynamic flux, the more fun and creativity we can enjoy.

Live there

The ancient texts describe many effects of a long-term practice. Indeed, it is frequently stated that for one who has conquered the surface mind, worldly concerns over things such as heat and cold, honour and dishonour, are no longer felt — such is the tranquillity attained[87].

In chapter four, I mentioned that a result of *prāṇāyāma* and *kumbhaka* practice was the sense of my thoughts existing further away from me, and that I possessed the new ability to wave them away before they fully reached me. As those mental effects of *yoga* became established, I also noticed an analogous lack of attachment in the physical. When I had a symptom like a sore throat — the unmistakeable start of a cold, I would anticipate falling sick the next day. But the next day nothing at all was wrong. I felt complete health. Just as I had habituated the waving away of undesired thoughts in my periphery, I was now seemingly waving away an undesired virus after giving it a brief glance.

With *yoga* and the cessation of unthinking mechanical attachment, scattered and ancillary things do not "stick to you" as much; you don't automatically grab every little thought or air-borne droplet that comes your way.

[87] Bhagavad Gītā 6.7

Your sense of the central pillar of energy becomes brighter, and relative distance from the material world increases, and this gives you a heightened experience of purposeful will. Attractions and aversions remain, but they feel optional and carry less sting. There are new and interesting places to visit that hold a greater allure.

Yoga can induce eerie physical sensations. Recall that when you go far up a physical mountain or a sky-scraper, the air pressure changes and there is a distinctly heady feeling — the perception of sound and space changes. Similarly, the spiritual mountain journey can present a proximal quality, as though you are up high on a precipice. A sense of shifting, a wobble here and there, shrinking and expanding.

Ultimately, when you shut your eyes, you ought to be able to go straight into subtle consciousness. Where imagery used to only be visible during sleep or after several minutes in meditation, now you can see it any time you like. You have uncovered more of yourself. Your unconscious is becoming conscious. All can come to light, and it is more enjoyable and helpful than suppression. This is the evolution beyond genetics.

The burning bed

There is an old Indian story of a person with a mango seed in their head. It is the principal *karmic* seed. If it is nourished or entertained, then it sprouts and spreads into the body, rooting and creating many related thoughts, a continuous supply of distraction.

To burn the seed of *karma* one must identify it and expose it to the spiritual air above, rather than watering it with activity. Awake and attentive, not pushing it away, not satisfying it. There it remains unmanifest, unresolved, exposed to all the possibilities and choosing none. The temptation to act is a doomed impulse to make it go away. But if it is acted upon, a chain of cause and effect will commence. Instead, pause and expose it to the elements. Wait, and it will not take root.

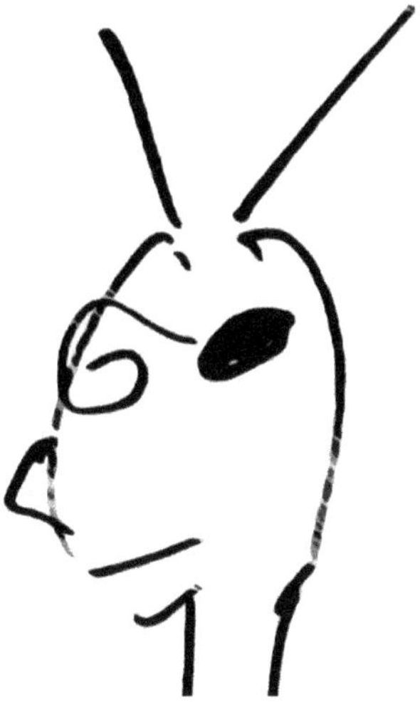

We have to open the top of our skull and become used to feelings of unbearable potential and uncertainty. Be willing not to ameliorate our desires, but to keep them unbearably open. This suspense fuels us, and we become a far more efficient and graceful channel for the spiritual.

Will you be able to handle the infinite consciousness yourself, alone, or will you need to create other people to talk to? Will the surface mind be able to cope with the transcendent, will it know and trust that all it needs to do is be still and watch? Or will it be unable to resist interrupting the flow by attaching and chattering?

You need to be able to lay in bed of *turīya*[88] at night knowing that every single thing in the material world that you derive comfort from is unstable and non-solid, somewhat absurd and illusory. All these things are temporary, as is your physical body — a constantly changing energetic form playing upon your own eternal screen of consciousness.

Laying there, in that fire of awareness, the seeds of *karma* are burned.

---

[88] Yoga Tārāvalī *śloka* 26

Compulsive or habitual action is called *prārabdha*, referring to complex linkages of cause and effect. If, in any moment, you act because you **cannot resist** it, then you are under control of *prārabdha karma.*

If, on the other hand, you easily see equality and neutrality in everything, the joy and the pain in both acting and not acting, then you have the mountaintop perspective. If you then choose to act, and you do so according to the urging of your inner authority, discernible by the quality of pure glee and innocent curiosity, then it is done in the service of your higher Self. This is the free will of the supervising *ātman*, as Śaṅkara says. The usual mode of action is diminished or destroyed altogether[89]. When you accommodate the thrilling energy and know it as your true Self, an optimally adaptive and unbounded intelligence called *buddhi* is found.

Again, I will draw your attention to the likelihood of forgetting all of this in the next instant, and the need to adopt a strategy to reduce the time between occurrences of remembering. This is why we schedule a regular *yoga* practice, and cultivate communities of people who are similarly keen. This is also why people collect triggers in the form of affirmations, trinkets, reminders.

Instantaneity

There is one more thing to note: our observed biology and the classical view of physics feature the notion of gradation. That is, the sun moves across the sky gradually, electrons orbit nuclei in a smooth arc, plants grow in stages, muscles become strong over time as we train them, buckets of water fill linearly, and so forth. But the reality is different.

Multi-dimensional reality — popularly called the multiverse — is **probabilistic** in nature. This means it can appear to operate by chance, and that the we measure the **likelihood** of things, rather than a straightforward path. All scenarios are played out in an infinite array of universes, and we

---

[89] Aparokṣānubhūti *śloka* 98

as conscious agents identify with this or that scenario at any perceivable moment in the human experience of time.

Our experience of gradation results from deliberately limiting our view, pretending not to see in other directions. Recall the story of humanity through *sanātan dharma* from chapter three. The longer the people stayed in the linear sandpit playing, the more forgetting occurred, knowledge of their true existence faded, and the truth slipped out of reach.

Our quest is to learn to move from scenario to scenario without so many tiny iterations, and the human brain is a fabulous vehicle to explore this. Brains are set up as deeply interconnected networks, just like computers. As we know from experience in the apparent external world, computers can be flashed with information in one single operation — so it is with brains.

You do not have to move gradually in a line from one state to another. You might think that you do, and you might have experiences that seem to confirm the belief that everything happens incrementally, that good things must be earned, that habits are hard to break, and that your mood is dependent on factors outside of your control.

But it does not have to work that way. A measure of evidence can be seen when a sudden thing happens in life, a positively or negatively received shock or event. There is an instantaneous change to your whole state of mind. There is no slow, gradual progression to feeling happy when you win the lottery, for example — you feel happy instantly.

On the other hand, physical sense organs and the personality connected to them are limited to sequential increments of space and time. Surface mind forgets easily and is flummoxed very quickly, so it prefers slow and measured movements. It relies on habits and a sense of certainty that is enabled by the explicit rules of materiality. But this is a distorted implementation of consciousness.

The mode of consciousness is "random access" and it can switch from one state to any other state in any moment. The belief that the next state must closely resemble the current one is artificial and unnecessary. You do not have to rewind or fast forward the tape to go to a different state; you simply identify the state you want and then "click" — go there.

This idea is reflected in the analogy of a **screen** of consciousness as the Indians tend to present it. Imagine a screen with many small pixels which you nonetheless view altogether at one moment. Compare this to the similar but very linear analogy of a **stream** of consciousness, which implies a sequence of many moments, requiring more time to access.

Indeed, Śaṅkara declares that true conscious control is the **instantaneous** arising of any state desired[90]. Intrinsically, we know that ideas come from somewhere strange and oblique. We know that if the surface mind were truly in charge, we would be in a lot of trouble. The ruler we have appointed appears untrustworthy and incomplete. We sense that we are not seeing the full picture, and this creates anxiety.

Your higher consciousness is not limited by tasks and time-frames. It is always ready to expose us to secrets in perfect timing, and to provide good ideas to run with. Take a deep breath — suspend your breath — interrupt the holding patterns of the babbling intellect. Let it assume its appropriate place as an implement, not a king. Reduce the throttling effect of the surface mind, with its narrow scope that allows only a mild seeping of creative ingredients into daily life.

---

[90] Aparokṣānubhūti *śloka* 125

Overflow

Open the floodgates and allow the overflow called *manonmanī* to occur[91].

As touched on in chapter six, you may imagine a handful of rivers that run roughly alongside each other. To move from one river to the other, in linear reality, requires back tracking from your position in the current river, up to a junction, and then down another river.

Now imagine a more radical approach where you increase the overall flow of water significantly in all rivers, you open the tap at the source. The water level rises across all rivers until they are overwhelmed and become one single body of water. Now you can go sideways, anywhere, at any time, no need to back-track. You have integrated the rivers; you have invoked the state of *manonmanī*. In the same way you can feel however you want, any time you want. You can flash your brain computer with any program desired.

Truly, the main thing you need to succeed at this is to simply be told that you can! A little practice may be required to wrestle the beliefs of the personality and make those new vistas available. Attain personal proof that relaxation and day-dreaming are necessary for optimal functioning — prudent investments which attract your desired states more effectively than trying to orchestrate every little step in a mechanical fashion.

This is important. If you will only allow yourself to feel better when material circumstances have arranged themselves favourably in a manner that "proves" to the intellect that danger has passed, or that you have "earned" what you desire, you may be waiting forever!

---

[91] Yoga Tārāvalī *śloka* 17

The surface mind cannot see the future; it can only chatter about what has already happened. If it does not know about the future-modifying functions of creative intention, then it will **never feel safe**.

The image in the mirror will only smile back to you when you smile first.

Create your world in ways that seem audacious. Be bold. Change the shape of the body, the length of muscles, physical skills and abilities. Feel like a different person. Reinvent yourself regularly. Change the negative fantasies that play in the mind to their exact opposite, use your imagination to flip your long-held beliefs — just to see if you can do it.

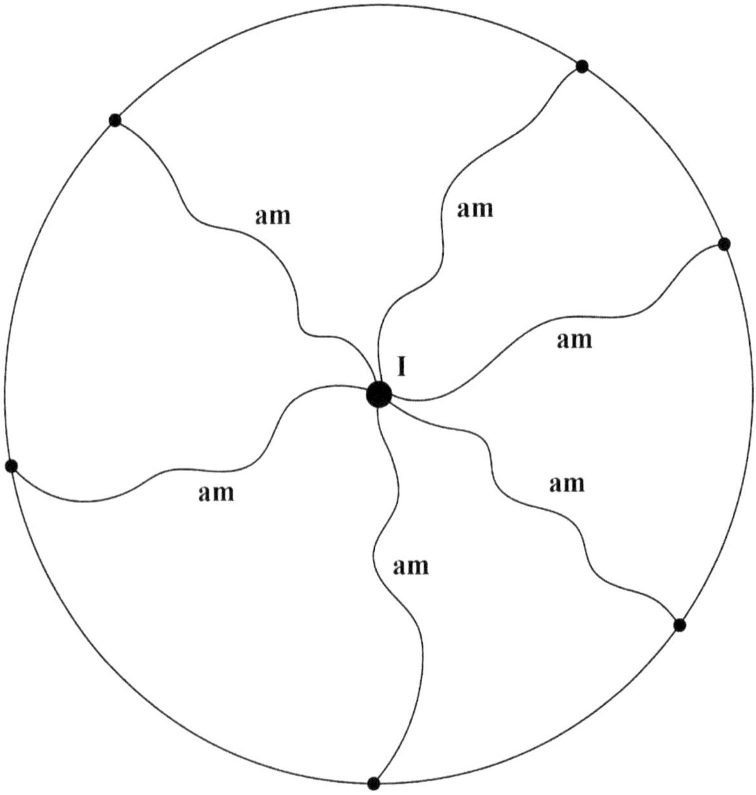

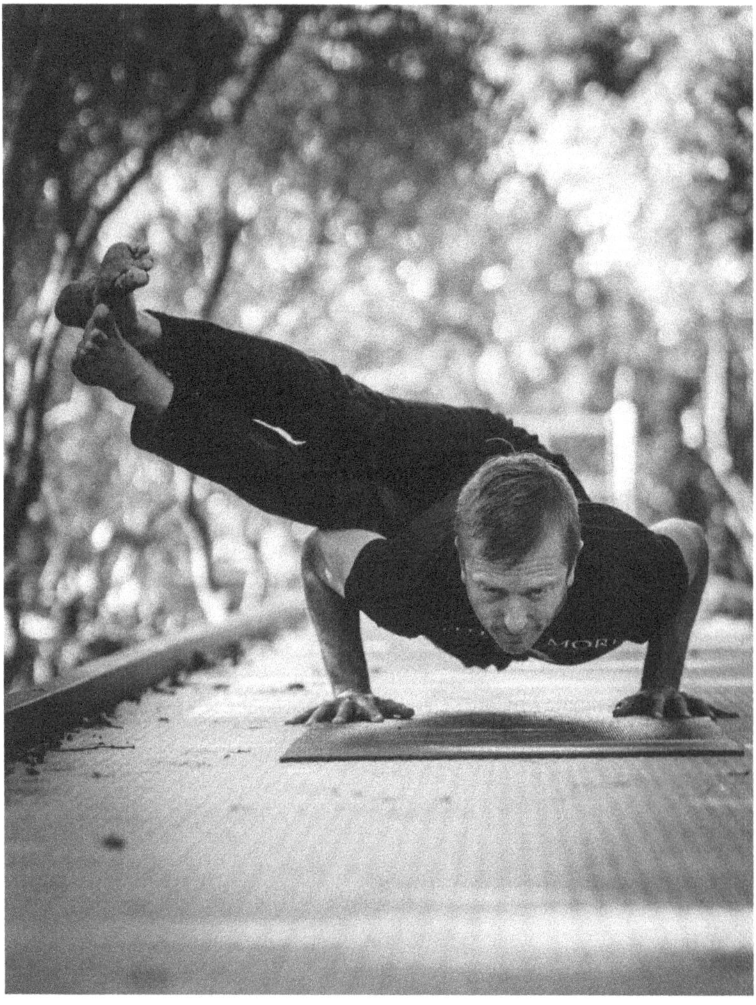

Photo credit: Dean Abraham

9

MOVE INTO DEEPER YOGA

"Even when the mind wavers and the eyes drift idly, the highest yoga has an uninterrupted course. There is nothing beyond this and nothing more conducive of doing good than this yoga. This science and knowledge should be made available to those devoted students who seek profundity, and protected from those who would be careless."

– Brahma Vidya Upanishad

The transformation of *yoga* occurs so gradually it is often unnoticed by the practitioner. Many times, a student's growth is pointed out by others before they themselves recognise it. A common effect, for example, is the frequent demonstration of better decision-making in tense situations — being "the calm one". The receipt of positive feedback from peers like this, along with the natural unfolding of new interests and curiosities, encourages us to keep moving along the path of inclusivity and honesty, as is our natural desire in life.

Restraints and observances

This brings us to the original Ashtanga Yoga of Patañjali, literally "eight-limbed" *yoga*, with each limb representing a stage along the path to *samādhi*. It is the journey to a naturally psychic and expansive life, starting with the basics and stretching right up to the mountaintop.

Limbs number one and two are *yama* and *niyama*, meaning behavioural controls and observances — the definition of the word "ethics". Limbs three and four are *āsana* and *prāṇāyāma*, and the rest are subtle processes of *pratyāhāra*, *dhāraṇā*, *dhyāna*, and finally *samādhi*. These rungs form a ladder known as *rājā yog*a — royal *yoga*, as it leads to the crown *cakra*, called *sahasrāra*.

The first two controls (*yama*) are the most important. They are: *satya* (truth), and *ahimsā* (non-violation). They can be reflected in a statement:

In each moment, seek to know your strongest inclination, that which evokes the strongest feeling of personal interest and virtue. Wholeheartedly pursue those actions that truly excite you in every moment unless it seems like a violation, according to your conscience.

Understanding this is the first step to reclaiming your inner authority and placing trust in your conscience. Your innate sense of right and wrong is to be energised, relied upon, and developed. By doing this, we unravel the doubt and guilt that has been imposed by religions that postulate we are all born sinners. Equally, we seek to undo the negative effects of an exclusively materialistic scientific culture which posits that we are all high-functioning apes who would revert to murdering each other, given the chance.

Just as you are the ultimate scientist in your life, so too you are the prime ethicist. We each have a conscience, regardless of the cultures in which we operate. This is a universal sense of right and wrong, an impulse for good, which we can trust above all else.

You can believe your own perceptions, and you can trust your ability to learn from actions and evolve. Humankind is intelligent and perceptive. We are civil. We created civilisation itself! Understand the validity of your authority over yourself, internalise the locus of control.

Through *yoga* you develop interoception and feel more keenly the effects of various kinds of food, exercise, and recreation on your body. You will naturally make better decisions based on this feedback loop. When people repress their pain, they are more likely to allow others — and the planet — to suffer too. In order to repress pain, you must segregate a part of yourself and then hide it from view. In order to hurt another creature, you must remove the living creature from your experience and hide its suffering from view. Beliefs like "it's every man for himself" push people in this disintegrative direction, which is a slippery slope to self-fulfilling justifications of negative behaviour.

On the other hand, when you deeply feel the effects of kindness, you will express that instead. When you understand that seemingly external people are contained within your own consciousness, you will be more inclined to love them and treat them well. A survivalist mindset transforms into natural compassion and altruism.

Those people exist within you! Hurting others **makes no sense**.

This is the metaphysical perspective on "self-love". In *yoga*, self-love is a practice of collecting, piece-by-piece, the fragments of yourself that are located on various isolated parts of the mountain face, and bringing them to light, bringing them into clear view. No dark corner of yourself goes un-examined. Self-love is the expression of infinitely expanding interest in the wellbeing of all of your Self.

Yoga will help you pin down what truly interests you, what arouses passion or evokes joy and excitement. Your awareness of this is a benefit to yourself and others. It is crucial to hear and see the Self, and all of the tones, messages, visions, and ideas that fly by your awareness. As this unfolds, it then becomes just as important to trust and act on them. These skills logically then become the over-arching pursuit in life.

Ancient texts

For students who have grown up on the standard diet of the Patañjali Yoga Sūtras, it is useful to know that there are alternate presentations of the same principles. This helps us check the tendency that we reviewed in chapter three to freeze good ideas into rigid dogma. The Yoga Sūtras are just one compilation of the teachings, which have existed for a long time, transmitted by many teachers all across the greater Himalayan areas. Teachers are bound to have different processes.

Upanishads and other texts from the canon present slightly different maps of *yoga*. Many of them present a number of limbs or stages, and of those there are variations of the number of limbs and their orders, and slightly different details. They all represent a coherent path to reaching the mountain top. For example, Śaṅkara presents fifteen stages of *yoga* in Aparokṣānubhūti, which includes the familiar *yama*, *niyama*, etc, and also includes as limbs *dṛṣṭi*, *bandha* and others[92].

In Mandala Brahman Upanishad, we find the familiar eight limbs, but there are different *yama* and *niyama*, compared to those Patañjali cites. They include the conquest of distress and craving, overcoming feelings of heat and cold in the body, adherence to the path of knowledge and the teacher who can impart it, deliberate enjoyment of the bliss that is beyond sense gratification, invocation of gratitude and contentment, making time to practice, and so forth.

The effectiveness of these principles and tools are clear for us to see. The evidence is in the community of practitioners — with people brightening up, moving through vicissitudes deftly, and actively making time for health and happiness. *Yoga* self-perpetuates as a result of the good feeling it provides. It is a good feeling that is particularly sustainable too, when taught in the Mysore style environment, which allows individuals to reach the pinnacle of *yoga* at their own pace.

---

[92] Aparokṣānubhūti *śloka* 100 - 125

The ancient texts of Indian metaphysics have a lot to offer. The questions we are currently asking, in modern scientific and philosophical discourse, are the same questions *yogin*-s were asking long ago, long before our sophistications and technology.

The texts are usually quite short and yet contain a great deal of information. Sanskrit is akin to a compressed or compiled language. Aphorisms were recorded on palm leaves using a bare minimum of space, and they are bereft of excessive flair or prosaic accoutrements. It was expected that a knowledgeable teacher would understand and draw out their meaning, embellishing the phrases for students to understand.

When studying, you must seek things that are **personally important and interesting**, those topics that feel fascinating. Recall that *ānanda*, spiritual excitation and bliss, is your compass. Keep following that feeling as it changes as well — you may feel elevated in regard to a topic one day and another the next. Beware the old habit of choosing one thing and running with it permanently, even when it has fulfilled its purpose. If you keep listening and selecting, *ānanda* will be continuous.

As familiarity with the Sanskrit language increases and the concepts clarify and are reinforced by experience, the texts magically come alive. It is wonderful to expose yourself, in a practical manner, to material written long ago by masters who were thinking along the same lines.

Straight translations from Sanskrit to English, those devoid of commentaries by modern authors, are powerful to absorb. It is usually necessary to read commentaries for a while, as you acclimatise yourself. In time, you may extricate yourself from the baggage of modern labels. For example, the English word "God" really ought not be used in any translation. **We** invented that word and **we** packed it solid with our own religious dogma. I have seen that word planted in translations in numerous contexts where other words as varied as "principle", "centre", "substrate", and "will" are more suitable. It is not appropriate to associate beautifully elaborate ancient Sanskrit terms with anything resembling a vengeful, bearded man in the sky. When studying, it is best to form an understanding on a fresh slate.

Āsana is inducement

A strong and regular, self-paced *āsana* practice is one of the greatest gifts that a human can give to themselves. It stokes *bhāvana* — aspiration and persistence — with which anything can be achieved.

It delivers freedom from bodily disturbance. Freedom in the body means feeling loose and indestructible, resilient and unbounded, able to balance, walk up mountains, do cartwheels in the park, throw children into the air, and catch them again without a second thought.

Āsana also delivers freedom from mental disturbance. Freedom in the mind is a can-do attitude, reinforced by innumerable instances of having overcome personal challenge.

When taught in a Mysore style environment, *āsana* teaches you to keep getting up, to keep resetting your intention and purpose, all under your own steam. It helps you recognise your own authorship and resilience. It trains you to keep joining the state of flow, over-and-over, every day.

It teaches you how to enjoy and sustain the slippery states of exaltation that we all feel from time-to-time. It teaches you how to bring them in and live with them. It fuels your natural state of wonder, correcting physical and energetic imbalances, allowing you to radiate positivity like a sun, influencing those in your proximity.

People feel good just being around you, they feel good after you have left, and they may even feel good when you are **about to enter** the room.

In this way, become a *yoga* student rather than *yoga* consumer.

Minister your mood

Control your thoughts. Minister your mood. Sit with a choice, feel both, and choose the one that feels good. This is natural meditation, actively using your higher consciousness in the world.

It is a gift to understand that you have abstract inner states and that they exist at all times, and can be experienced **at all times**. You are the ultimate will. There is no other. You can ascertain all of your Self, all of the time, and thus be the total creator of your experience.

Simply put, with a little attention, you can control the plants that germinate in your garden, you can control what ingredients are simmered in your saucepan — why not choose what to illuminate in your mind? Accessing the desired *pratyaya* is simply about discovering how, rather than labouring at the process. We tend to assume that everything takes time, and that good things are out of reach and need to be earned. However, you can access any state from any other state.

You can select a nicer state from the array of options available in your memory and imagination, and then activate it. In the early days, it can seem more plausible to journey from an undesired state such as anger, to a full and blissful state via a more neutral state. If doing this, one must remember to keep going through the neutrality, out the other end. Just remember that neutrality is not the end goal — it is a rest point.

Initially, you could feel a bit daft, as though you are fooling yourself. Or, you could feel frustrated because it's not working. That is okay, be persistent. Doubt and frustrations work their way up to be seen and transformed. They perform a function — don't give up in the process.

The current culture has a strong belief that we cannot rule ourselves, that our minds are unreliable and we need governments and studies and churches to look after us. The concept of the unconscious or subconscious mind is a symptom of this, delegating parts of ourselves to concealed areas. It is a game that has been played for a very long time, and we can choose another way. We can trust ourselves again.

Trust the feeling of innocent curiosity and playfulness that has accompanied you throughout your life. It never went away. It gently taps you on the shoulder. Bring it in, allow it to expand and sit in every pore of your being. It raises your consciousness, it spirals upwards, affecting every moment and every particle, and that includes the apparent other people in existence. If you can let this perspective reside within you — if you can reside within it, you will have discovered the most valuable trick of consciousness. It is called *dhyāna* — a constant stream of remembrance. The seat is always there, atop the mountain, waiting for you to slip into position.

Life flashes before your eyes

A well-known anecdote is that when a person dies, or nearly dies, their life flashes before their eyes. The vantage from the top of the mountain is the same — you can see your entire life. Not so much reliving it in a linear sequence, rather, you have clear access to it all as a witness.

Everything makes sense when you see all the components as one whole thing — one event containing themes, actors, and places. Instead of seeing the movie frame-by-frame, you see the whole reel and can navigate it at will. Transcend linear time and acquire spontaneous access to anything you like. Consider the familiar musing of how lovely it would be to have both the wisdom of age and the innocence of youth at once — well here it is. *Yoga* offers this as a regular state of being.

You are the one unified being that is self-contained and omnipresent, while also existing as numerous diverse pieces. The Indians refer to this as *viśiṣṭādvaita* — the one and the many, formless non-duality along with the forms and attributes of duality. This is the final teaching and it is best delivered via disarming paradox, known as *acintyabhedābheda*, the inconceivable co-existence of both one-ness and difference.

You are the focal point that traverses the mountain. You can play within the world of appearances, and still access the mountaintop. You can have a life of creative experience, with all the freshness of first-times and sense pleasure, while remaining clairvoyant and able to sculpt circumstances according to your own sense of good story-telling.

You are a comet

To put it another way — you are a comet. You are *śiva* at the head, piloting it through space. You are *avante garde*, the leading-edge, navigating the thrillingly unmanifest uncertainty. The tail of the comet consists of material effects, fragments of history, objects and particles.

When you wish to create something in the phenomenal world, do it first on the top of the mountain, at the head of the comet. It is much easier there; momentum is on your side and the details look after themselves. Rather than changing one thousand small things in the material life, persistently foster the essential state that aligns with your desire, ahead of time.

As you reach into the future, be at this leading edge. Be the visionary. Everything you know resides in your imagination, so act in that way. Creativity abounds in proportion to the degree of attention invested. Uncover what you want and focus your attention on how it feels. See how events become injected with your feelings. Hold in your mind the *pratyaya* of choice. Allow thoughts and actions to flow from this intent.

It is right to rebel against cynicism and assumptions that were waved through without explanation. Informed consent includes being responsible for all of your creations, and being eager to venture beyond the comfort zone of the ordinary material debris in favour of the exciting fluidic activity at the head. All the great perspectives and all the desired states are always available. In any moment, even if you feel separate and lost, the higher vantage is still there — you just have to remember it and go there.

Deva worship

Spiritual sacrifice is not about performing ceremonies, being a martyr to a cause, or affecting a pretence of spirituality. These things remove you from a natural, organic, playful life of innocent mischief. The true sacrifice is disrupting the addiction to materiality, and instead tending to the garden of visualisations, tones, and ideas. It is called sacrifice because there is a giving up of something that you hold close — your ingrained routines.

The purpose of Indian deities, *deva*, is to house collections of *pratyaya* so that they can be quickly accessed. They are configurations of ideas that serve human beings who wish to evolve. They are placeholders, handy entities that offer non-verbal intentions, geometries, relationships, metaphors. They are there to rouse you toward your memory of your own idealised visions, moods, and concepts of being.

You are a constantly changing energetic form, being refreshed in every moment, and you can choose your ingredients in every moment.

Use deities to load sets of ingredients that are relevant in the moment. They are a configuration of ingredients in consciousness, and it is completely valid to have this approach with other figures, other gods, other teachers in history, musicians, ancestors, leaders of society, animals, and fictional characters. Any symbol at all, really.

What matters is how it makes you feel and act.

Upon seeing the mythology and ritualism of **modern** Hinduism, you might summarily discard the wealth of Indian thought as yet another religious culture fused with monarchy and capitalism. But this would be a mistake. Organised religion has been exposed as a power-hungry controller of minds, and we can take back the power of gesture and symbolism, to help us remember the goal, to remember who we are.

The enormity of metaphysical insight developed over thousands of years by those seers in the Indus Valley has begun to be made available to us only recently, through translations. Do not dismiss it as religion in order to go about materialist life. See instead, those deities pregnant with meaning, containing ideas of the highest value, ready to be invoked.

I am *śiva*, sitting atop the mountain of my vast Self. I have access to all memory and ideations, all poise and patience, all willpower and trust in the ecstatic and inevitable realisation of truth in a way that is so interesting and invigorating that, given the chance, I would find the choice to be reborn 1000 more times hard to resist.

To remember these positive feelings and your power to select them, is the purpose of spirituality and all spiritual tools. It is the purpose of deities, poetry, photos, trinkets, souvenirs, chants, gestures, and rituals. They all help you remember and reorient towards a desired state. For a Westerner, the simple use of prayer-hands, *añjali mudrā*, and words like *namaste* can be powerful — adopting an attitude that has existed long before our own culture, peeking into our distant ancestry.

I understand and acknowledge that you exist in me and I exist in you, that we are nominally separate facets of one sole being.

A man glances at a photo of his family on his desk and he recalls holidays past, and holidays to come, and it helps him put his crowded inbox into perspective.

A man glances at a statue of *śiva* sitting on a mountain with light pouring into his skull from outer space, and he remembers that he is the sole controller of his interpretation of reality, and that it is up to him to select an elevated mood, and enjoy an idealised life in intimate harmony with all in his proximity.

In the culture of Mysore style teaching, and in Ashtanga Vinyasa Yoga, we have various affectations to use as reminders. There are opening and closing chants, photographs of revered teachers, statues of deities on an altar at the front of the room, and many similar things.

Students will often turn themselves around head-to-toe as they rest at the end of practice, so that they do not show their feet to the deity, as a symbol of deference. If this feels good to you, by all means join in, if not, perhaps something else.

When you have finished your *yoga* practice in the studio, you might take a moment to quietly sing the closing chant, called *maṅgala mantra.* Let the novelty and gravity of such gestures enliven you and your community.

We are all one single existence,
and we are all diversity and individuality.

eko 'ham bahu śyāma – I am one and I become many.
aham brahmasmi – I am the ultimate reality.
hare krishna – I am the cosmic person.

240

Epilogue

Calamitous events like the coronavirus pandemic can serve us. **Humanity needs rest.** We are given a time-out, an opportunity to rest and then make decisions with more clarity about how we want to conduct ourselves.

People are prone to mechanical and robotic behaviours, addicted to the sugar and drama treadmill. If we just keep battling on, pushing our bodies, and bullying the big spherical body that we live upon, we'll get a slap. It is better to consciously make time for relaxation and contemplation, as humble and respectful students of nature. When we evolve spiritually, the world we embody becomes more beautiful. Gregor again notes:

> *"Inner freedom can never be attained by following a set of rules, a formula. Freedom is awareness. Any rules will be used by the mind and ego to build a new prison. The rejection of all rules, however, is just a new formula. The way out is, rather than through creating yet another set of rules, turning around and becoming aware of that which needs no regulation, that which breathes life into everything, and therefore cannot be opposed to life. When that is seen, great compassion for all living beings arises spontaneously from the heart and does not have to be imposed by the mind. Then we become living ethics, whereas before we tried to simulate life through a dead set of rules. Ethics can never replace mystical insight, but they clear the way to getting there."*[93]

[93] Maehle, G., "Samadhi: The Great Freedom" (Crabbes Creek: Kaivalya Publications 2015)

When nerves get saturated, the muscles get knotted, the endocrine system works overtime and it becomes difficult to concentrate and regulate emotions. Stress supresses the immune system, creates inflammation, and tightens the body. So, lay down and rest.

Nature heals itself very quickly when the source of stress abates. Allow the rivers in your own body a bit of rest. Drink clear water. Do lots of stretching and sun salutations. Do far, far less social media. Spend more time with yourself in silence, acknowledge and feel any angst, and it will pass. Share deep things with people, rather than gossip. Share your love of nature, your dreams, your vision for heaven on earth. Share your silence too, your comfort with non-physical communication.

Transform your anxiety. After all, it proves you are capable of intense concentration and such vivid imagination that your body exhibits signs of actually experiencing the event! Even your heart rate and blood pressure are affected. Use this power to induce the states you prefer.

Make time to pursue creative visualisation. Do it the way elite sports-people do it, by going into imagination and playing and replaying a fantasy in your mind. Practice feeling what it is like, how good it feels, acting it out. Go into specifics — actually experience it. Your brain is a programable filter, and it will hone in on anything you want it to. Left to its devices you will experience a mixed bag at best. Instead, train it to show you what you want to see, through the process of "make-believe". You are already doing this **all of the time**, so take control of the tool.

If it feels silly — that's okay. Keep going. After a while you will not have to force the positive aspiration as much, it takes on a life of its own — just as anxiety used to. Serendipitous and useful information appears spontaneously. Visions grow and they impinge upon your experience. The act of imagining can become as fun as experiencing the event itself.

While sitting with eyes closed, dive into the fantasy with as much zeal as you can muster. Regularly spend 10 minutes seeing and interacting with full emotional expression. Be self-assured and content, unflinching in your certainty that the intention is instantly transmitted far and wide, flooding into the countries of the world and the galaxies of the universe.

Watch as your waking and sleeping experiences become tuned in the direction of your noble aspiration. Allow the fantasy to be released from the proximity of your skull — the false perimeter that you have now shed.

All places are inside your consciousness, there is nothing bigger than you. As you experience your physical body to be **inside** your consciousness, and stretch out into the rest of your Self, you may communicate far and wide in an instant, using the subtle language of tones, proto-linguistic forms, visions, and ideals. Your ordinary daily routine will become an adventure. Every moment contains an insight, a signpost, an opportunity to revere and reinforce your vision, and to receive help and opportunities out of left-field.

Do it. It's not corny — it's the way we create — we are dreamers. The dreams that we repeatedly invest with time and emotion become physical. If we get stuck dreaming about worst-case scenarios, then we are wasting our greatest tool, driving it into a ditch.

The effort you invest while practicing *yoga* pays dividends during your day. A vigorous and repetitive *āsana* practice is one of the best ways to deeply remind yourself amongst the various demands of worldly life.

Consciousness is the beginning and the end — it is the Garden of Eden. You are the ever-existing witness, you are the author, the scientist, the artist, the translator, the illustrator. You are the planetary canvas and the night sky. You are cosmic waves of unity, reflecting all potential and power in the form of past-present-future.

All information comes from you, to you.

You are playfully proving yourself, to yourself.

Flex and extend yourself in the direction of positive.

Salute the sun!

Glossary

abhyāsa — discipline, habit, drill

acintyabhedābheda — incomprehensible co-existence of multiplicity and unity, the paradox of there being a thing that is beyond numeration and yet contains numbered objects

advaita and *dvaita* — non-duality and duality

ājñā — command (centre of)

ākāśa — sky, atmosphere, space, ether

amanaska — without mind, no inner chatter

amṛta — ambrosia, nectar of eternality

anāhata — produced without physical action

añjali — reverence

annamaya — made of foodstuff, physical entity

anusandhāna — close inspection, investigation

āsana — seat, dwell, posture

asmitā — sense of personal identity

aṣṭāṅga — eight parts or members

ātman — character, essence, self

avadhūta — shaken off, agitated, discarded

avidyā — lack of knowledge, incomplete science

bandha — fasten, bind

bhakti — that which belongs to or is contained in anything else, succession, fondness

bhāga — component, phase, stage

bhagavan — glorious, prosperous, adorable one

bhastrikā — bag, bellows

bhāvana — producing, promoting, bringing about by faith

brahman — universal highest principle, the pervasive cause of causes, binding unity

buddhi — the faculty of awareness, wakefulness, attention, knowledge

cakra — wheel, disk

cikitsā — therapy, treatment

dhāraṇā — maintenance, steadfastness, concentration

dharma — works, character, virtue, decree, statute

dhyāna — profound attention, uninterrupted contemplation

dṛṣṭi — vision, focus

guṇa — quality, feature, attribute

guru — heavy, with gravity, significant teacher

gurukula — residence or community of the teacher

haṭha — with the use of physical effort or force

īśvara — master, ruler, king

jalandhara

kaivalya — absolute unity, perfect isolation

kāma —pleasure, gratification, sensuality

karma — action, work

kevala — alone, exclusive, simple, pure, unmingled

khecarī — one who flies through the atmosphere

kośa — container, envelope

kumbhaka — retain air as does a jar or pot

kuṇḍalinī — goddess power coiled like a snake

laya — melt, dissolve, absorb, rest

līlā — play, sport

manas — lowest part of the mind that bridges senses and rational thought

maṅgala — auspicious, prosperous

manonmanī — flooding of the mind

mantra — formula, design, plan, speech

māyā — phantom, apparition

mudrā — imprint, sign, attitude, token

mukha — mouth, face, surface, summit

mūla — base, source, root

mūrcchā — swooning, fainting

nāda — sounding, crying, roaring

nadī — river, conduit, hollow tube

namaste, namaskāra — greetings, salutations, reverence

pañca kośa — model of five increasingly subtle layers of being
prajñā — state of dreamless sleep
prakṛti — building blocks of the empirical material world
prāṇa — vital and life-giving air
prāṇāyāma — breath extension
prārabdha — work that has commenced
pratibhā — splendorous genius, flash of intelligence, audacious creativity
pratyāhāra — withdraw, retreat
pratyaya — thought, assumption, analysis, idea, notion
puruṣa — person, witness, principle of consciousness
rājā yoga — "royal" *yoga* that deals with mind and consciousness
rajas — passion, brimming zeal
ṛṣi — seer, sage, poet, ray of light
saccidānanda — the combination of all existence, knowledge, and bliss
sadhana —means, instrument, process
sahaja — innate, natural, birthright
sahasrāra — sun of a thousand rays
śaktipāt — instant bestowing of knowledge
samadarśin — neutral view of things
samasthiti — evenly centred position
saṃsāra — wandering though mundane cycles, metempsychosis
sanātan dharma — perpetual and ancient purpose
sattva — harmony found between two opposites, purity
śāmbhavī — born from bliss, that which is from Śiva
saṃyama — binding together the mind and an object
Śiva — the omniscient grace and will within all
śloka — verse, stanza
śodana — clearing up, correcting, sifting
sthirā — stable, fixed
sukha — happiness, delight
sūrya — sun, solar, deity of the sun
suṣumṇa — most gracious and stimulating artery or channel
sūtra — thread or string of aphorism

svarūpa — most true and complete form, handsome and pleasing

taijasa — dreaming state, endowed with light

tamas — inertia, lethargy

trāṭaka — fixing the eye on an object

turīya — the fourth state of consciousness that supervises waking, dreaming, and sleeping

uḍḍīyana — flying up, soaring

unmanī — no mindedness, trans-mental state

upaniṣad — to sit near to

ūrdhva — elevated, aloft, upwards

vāc — the principle of speech

vairagya — indifference, aversion, freedom from attachment

vāsanā — unconscious tendencies persisting by means of long-term memory

vijñānamaya — layer of being characterised by pure science, understanding, and wisdom

vinyasa — composition, connecting movements, ordered utterance

viṣaya — field, domain

viśiṣṭādvaita – pre-eminent form of integrative metaphysics, enhanced non-dualism

viṣṇu — the all-pervasive substance or principle

viveka — right discernment

yama and *niyama* — observances and restraints

yogin and *yoginī* — one who practices *yoga* (male and female)

Index

creativity
expression, 13, 97–98, 237
finding, 5, 15, 24, 60–61, 105, 117–118, 128, 212, 219, 224–225, 236–237, 244
in *yoga* practice, 12–13, 19–20, 97, 181
cycles of remembering and forgetting, 67, 272
cynicism, 110, 128, 202, 237

D

dancers, 71–72, 89
day-dreaming, 177, 208, 225
deities *(deva),* 238–240
devotion, 26–30, 54, 136–138, 195
dharma, 12. *see also sanātan dharma*
dhyāna, 87, 136, 230, 236
dialogue. *see also* speech
inner, 31, 40–47, 115–116, 131, 207, 212–215, 217, 220, xvii
with teacher, 19–20
disabilities, students with, 190–192
discipline, 172–173, 182, 187–188, 195. *see also abhyāsa*; *tapas*
dogmatism, 20, 44, 50–52, 59, 124, 183, 191, 232, 234
doubt, 118, 127, 161, 196, 202, 207, 213, 230, 234
dreams
dream consciousness, 91, 112–113, 130, 134–136, 138, 144, 146–148
and memory, 12–13, 109, 112, 115
when awake, 164, 208
dṛṣṭi, 144, 232
dualism, 127, 236. *see also* non-dualism
dvaita, 127
dvandva, 98. *see also* opposites

E

eight-limbed yoga (*aṣṭāṅga*), 114, 230, 232.
empathy, 2, 3, 30, 73, 100–101, 129, 158
enthusiasm, 25, 30–31, 63, 127, 168, 177, 188–189, 202, 214. *see also* aspiration

J

K

L

M

R

S

T

U

V

Milton Keynes UK
Ingram Content Group UK Ltd.
UKHW020903300424
441946UK00011B/909

9 780645 121100